In the Psychiat

Anthony Clare is Medical Director of St
Patrick's Hospital and Clinical Professor of
Psychiatry at Trinity College, Dublin.

ANTHONY CLARE

In the Psychiatrist's Chair

Mandarin

A Mandarin Paperback

IN THE PSYCHIATRIST'S CHAIR

First published in Great Britain 1992
by William Heinemann Ltd
This edition published 1993
by Mandarin Paperbacks
an imprint of Reed Consumer Books Limited
Michelin House, 81 Fulham Road, London SW3 6RB
and Auckland, Melbourne, Singapore and Toronto

Reprinted 1993

Copyright © Anthony Clare 1992
The author has asserted his moral rights

A CIP catalogue record for this title
is available from the British Library
ISBN 0 7493 1028 6

Printed and bound in Great Britain
by Cox & Wyman Ltd, Reading, Berks

To my friend and colleague Michael Ember who has taught me and many others so much and who, in addition to being a loyal friend, has been one of those professional broadcasters who have by virtue of their talent and integrity maintained and enhanced the reputation of BBC Radio 4 as one of the great radio networks in the world.

Contents

Arthur Ashe

Of the sixty plus interviews that I have undertaken since the series first started in 1982, is there one that I remember best? I am reluctant to pick one out because the truth is that I remember many of the interviews and for all sorts of reasons – the politician Edwina Currie telling me quite matter-of-factly of the break-up of her relationship with her father and his never speaking to her again, the novelist Susan Hill detailing the dreadful impact of a succession of miscarriages on her physical and mental state, the Bishop of London, Graham Leonard, admitting that on seeing a woman priest on the altar he might well feel an irresistible urge to go and put his arms around her, the pianist Vladimir Ashkenazy describing his mother's contempt for his circus entertainer father and her intense ambition that her young and talented son might be the internationally respected musician his father never would be, the black American writer Maya Angelou giving me a tough time when I used 'black' as an adjective to describe melancholic mood, the composer Sir Michael Tippett launching without delay into a frank and moving account of his homosexuality. And there are more, many more which made choosing the dozen that constitute the contents of this book so very difficult and so very arbitrary.

But there is one interview that I do recall with particular feeling and it is the one I had with Arthur Ashe in a radio studio in New York City. I did not start particularly auspiciously. When Ashe arrived I was instantly struck by his extraordinary composure, his cat-like grace, the ease with which he moved, the soft tone of his voice. It quickly became clear that he did not really know what the interview involved and he appeared somewhat disconcerted by the revelation that I was a psychiatrist. It was very subtly communicated – a steely edge creeping into his voice, a wary, watchful expression clouding his face. He listened carefully, respectfully, to my explanation of what I was about.

He then quickly relaxed and settled down but I had seen, however briefly, a hint of the emotions behind the impassive mask and the impressive control that he characteristically exercises. So it was not particularly surprising that the issue of emotional control surfaced repeatedly during our discussion. There were, though, other reasons. Arthur Ashe had won a remarkable victory in the Men's Singles Final at Wimbledon in 1975 by calmly and clinically out-foxing an increasingly aggressive and excitable Jimmy Connors. It was a thrilling contest between brain and brawn. (This provided a sweet irony for Ashe; in a part of the interview which was not broadcast, he regretted the tendency in America in the 1970s to see athletes in general as people with much brawn and little brain and black athletes in particular as people with even greater brawn and no brains at all). There was too the appalling Ashe family history of heart disease. Some argue that the high rates of high blood pressure and heart disease reported in black Americans are in part at least attributable to the inordinate control they struggle to exercise over negative feelings, feelings such as anger, resentment, frustration and rage. The American black, it is sometimes argued, is trapped between two competing stereotypes. He can act out the sterotype of the primitive African – Muhammed Ali deliberately, insolently, sardonically taunting whites with his calculated embodiment of their most extreme fantasies of the disinhibited black savage – or he can contain and repress his feelings risking the development of an over-compensating state of extreme control, feelings damned up inside an increasingly stressed and hypertensive body. Ashe appeared to many observers to personify the latter. It was not that he does not have emotions – he once walked off a court in a Masters tournament in Stockholm because he was fed up with the behaviour of his opponent Ilie Nastase but his demeanour remained impassive without a hint of his inner turmoil. So strong was Ashe's reputation for self-control that from time to time he would undergo a barrage of accusations of Uncle Tomism, of a desire to be a black surrogate version of a white man, from some radical blacks.

A second theme relates to Ashe's personal sense of death.

For Ashe this sense came early. When he was six, his grand-father died and shortly afterwards his own mother. While the tendency to personalise death occurs at all ages, it is most pronounced in children aged between five and ten. An obsession with death not uncommonly occurs in those who as children have had particular contact with it. Ashe denies obsession yet it is clear that he has a very intense, very intimate familiarity with death, is interested in cemeteries, morgues. Not surprising you might say of a man who, for all his athletic physique and talent, had two heart attacks and two cardiac operations before he reached forty. But Ashe admits to having been fascinated by death at an even earlier age. Nowadays all reasonably informed people are to varying extents involved in a permanent encounter with death. As Robert Kastenbaum and Ruth Aisenberg observe in their remarkable book *The Psychology of Death*[1], however engrossed we may be in our daily activities 'there lurks somewhere within us, ready for arousal, a complex of attitudes and anxieties based on the realization that any hour of any day could be doomsday.' Arthur Ashe encountered death, his mother's death, at six. He came face to face with his own mortality thirty years later. Laughingly he told me of a palm reader who insisted he had a long life-line but this man is no fool, no self-deceiver. He respects the relentless gene. 'I don't think I will live to the maximum.'

I write these words having just learned that Arthur Ashe has AIDS – that the blood transfused into his arteries and veins in July 1983 during his cardiac by-pass operation was contaminated with the HIV virus. His opening words in the interview he gave me now possess an eerie quality, his search in the lives of others for that one moment, that one event, that one experience 'when their life changed completely, they became what they're known for.' Since 1975 Ashe had been known as the first black man to win Wimbledon. Now he is known as a carrier of the world's most lethal infection. Soon he will be

[1] *The Psychology of Death*, Robert Kastenbaum and Ruth Aisenberg, Duckworth, London 1974

known as a major figure in the public campaign against the disease.

Arthur Ashe is a private man. He was extremely reluctant to publicise the fact that he had AIDS, pointing out at a press conference that he was not running for public office nor did he have share-holders to answer to. 'It is only because I fall under the dubious umbrella of public figure.' He argued that it should have been up to him to decide whether to reveal that he had AIDS. He certainly does not want the publicity that accompanies AIDS, the aura that surrounds the disease and the metaphors that encourage the ignorant and prejudiced to fulminate against sufferers. His decision to go public certainly constitutes one of those moments, those events which, in his words, change a person's life completely.

That is not to say that any one event actually forms any of us, least of all someone as talented, complex and subtle as Arthur Ashe. But if there is one such event in Ashe's life, then for me it remains his mother's death. In the last moments of the interview with me, he expressed a wish to meet his mother again and that she would hold him for a while, for a long time 'because I can't recall that ever having happened'. Ashe here expresses in his wish a link between birth and death, a link which the psychologist Sylvia Anthony, on the basis of interviewing children on the subject of death, suggested resulted from three meanings which children give death – death as separation or departure, death as sleep and death as going into a grave, coffin, earth and water.[1] The most common effect of death on children is of someone going away, for the departure that is death seems at first a departure like any other. My own seven-year-old son often talks of his grandfather, who died over two years ago, 'coming back to see us'. Anthony suggested that linking the concept of death with birth results in a belief that 'the actual pattern of life in time will be symmetrical with the symmetry suggested by the common aspects of birth and death as union with and separation from the mother'. Specu-

[1] *The Child's Discovery of Death*, Sylvia Anthony, Harcourt Brace and World, New York, 1940.

lation? Perhaps. But listen to Arthur Ashe – 'the boy in me, the little boy in me wonders if I will see my mother again, if I die that makes the spectre of dying more palatable.'

CLARE: Arthur Ashe was born on 10 July 1943 in Richmond, Virginia. His mother died, aged twenty-seven, of complications of high blood pressure and heart disease, when he was only six. And he and his younger brother were brought up by his father. Arthur Ashe started to play tennis as a seven-year-old, and aged seventeen won the United States National Juniors Indoor Championships. In 1968 he won the American Open Championships at Forest Hills and in 1970 won the Australian Open. In 1975 he became Wimbledon champion, crushing the hotly favoured Jimmy Connors in four sets. That same year he won the WCT finals in Dallas, beating Bjorn Borg. In addition to being one of the outstanding players of the 1970s, Arthur Ashe has played a major role in the reorganisation and development of the sport, being treasurer of the newly formed Association of Tennis Professionals in 1969 and its president in 1972. He was non-playing captain of the United States Davis Cup Team in the early 1980s. In 1979 Ashe suffered a serious heart attack and had to undergo by-pass surgery. His competitive tennis days ended. In July 1983, just short of his fortieth birthday, he underwent further open heart surgery. In the circumstances perhaps it's understandable that Ashe is a reflective man, with firmly held views on life, sport, politics and racism, views expressed clearly in his autobiography *Off the Court*, published in 1981. In that book I learned that Ashe's favourite reading is biography because he enjoys trying to find out what makes other people tick. What about yourself, I asked him, how do you feel about talking about what makes you tick?

ASHE: I don't mind it, er, too much. I don't feel any embarrassment over it. I am fascinated by what made other people what they are. In particular I'm looking for that one event in their life, that one moment, when their life changed completely, they became what they're known for or whatever, that breakthrough, that plateau that you reach. Almost everybody goes through that.

CLARE: And yours was what?

ASHE: Mine happened when I was ten years old, when I was playing on the courts next to my house in Richmond, Virginia. The tournament director of the Black College saw me playing during an idle moment when the courts weren't being used and from that moment on things changed. For instance, if I had been playing baseball during that time, if I'd been doing anything else at all, except being on that court where Dr Johnson could see me during that moment, and he had the wherewithal to take me even further than, I wouldn't have done anything else that I did later.

CLARE: So, in that sense that bears out what some people say about life, that its crucial moments are accidental ones?

ASHE: Yes, being in the right place at the right time. That has happened to me more than once and I always look for that in the biographies of other people.

CLARE: Yes. Other times it's happened to you would include when?

ASHE: Oh, I've been in the right place at the right time several times, even during my heart attacks, in '79, on July 31st, there just happened to be a doctor at the next court, on the next court where I was playing and had this difficulty and he saw me. He didn't know me personally but saw I was having some difficulty and he stopped what he was doing and came over and asked me a couple of questions and then rushed me to the hospital.

CLARE: That was here in Manhattan?

ASHE: Yes. As I found out later, the younger you are when you have a heart attack the higher the fatality rate, particularly if you don't do something immediately. It's the stalling, it's the denial of having the heart attack that proves fatal to quite a few people who die before they get to the hospital. You have to get to the hospital quickly. If you get there and you're still breathing you're in pretty good shape. But most people die because they say, 'I'm not having a heart attack, it's heartburn or indigestion or something.' So, again, I was in the right place at the right time.

CLARE: When it happened to you, did you likewise feel, it's indigestion, it's heartburn? I ask you that because you had and have written about quite an extensive family history of heart disease.

ASHE: Yes, which I didn't really appreciate until my experience. If I had, if even my personal doctor had paid more attention to my family history, not withstanding my athleticism, I should have been checked out more thoroughly.

CLARE: When you mentioned the events, those crucial events that you look for in others, do you look at it in terms of your life as a tennis player?

ASHE: No, actually I don't. I don't really look at it in terms of my life as a tennis player because very few other people are noted for something that they do temporarily. A professional athlete's time as a professional athlete is limited and when he or she retires, he or she is still very young. So I don't look at it in terms of my life as a tennis player. I look at it in terms of my life as a series of things I will do, tennis being just one of them.

CLARE: What I was getting at was that there are events that determine how these phases develop and of course an earlier event to the event on the court was the death of your mother, when you were quite a young boy.

ASHE: Yes, I still can't figure that one out. I have problems with that even today.

CLARE: Because?

ASHE: I don't know. I also learned in talking to an analyst, that because I just got so intrigued with it, that's probably the wrong word, I was so troubled by it, I could never explain it fully. He says that's very typical of young boys who lose their mothers at an early age, to have trouble dealing with it all the rest of their life.

CLARE: How much do you remember about her?

ASHE: Not even remotely as much as I would like to remember. I would like to know a hell of a lot more about her but an analyst also said that when that happens, typically a young boy just blocks it out. Not only do you block out memories of experiences with your mother but you block out everything else with it. So I have difficulty remembering anything that happened before I was six, anything at all, because I blocked everything out.

CLARE: You remember, though, her death.

ASHE: Yes, yes, I remember, I remember her, the last time I saw her alive. I remember the day of her funeral because I did not go.

CLARE: Because?

ASHE: My father asked me if I wanted to go and I said, I don't know why I said, 'No,' but I said no. I think also it was because my grandfather, my father's father had died less than a year earlier. So here was my father losing two very close people to him within the span of one year. But I also remember an aunt of mine crying hysterically at my grandfather's funeral and I remembered not liking it. I remember thinking to myself I wish she would stop and I thought maybe if there was going to be more of that sort of behaviour at my mother's funeral then I don't want to go.

CLARE: Does that trouble you now?

ASHE: That I said no? No, no, that doesn't trouble me at all, because I can't hold myself responsible for making the – quote unquote – 'right decision' when I'm six years old, especially if my father gives me the option. No, what troubles me is just that I would like to have remembered more. I can't remember my mother ever having held me or anything like that. I can't even fathom that, and I would like to fathom it but I can't. It's troubling, I'll tell you. It's very troubling, but then again I was made to understand very easily that – hey – it happens to everybody who loses a mother at an early age.

CLARE: In what way did it have an influence, do you think, on you?

ASHE: I have a very large family on both sides, Black American culture is built upon an extended family, informally anyway. My aunts tell me that I became very withdrawn and I myself know that I retreated into the world of sports and books and I guess that's where I have stayed ever since.

CLARE: You mention about the culture being an extended family culture. Does that mean that your family even now, the extended family, they're very important and that's where you find your support?

ASHE: Yes, yes, it was important that there were enough other family members around to make, to retain the sense of family, of thinking that you still belong to a family and also I gained a very healthy appreciation of my father's willingness to take on the role of father and mother too.

CLARE: He was quite a young man when this happened.

ASHE: Yes, yes, he was not thirty.

CLARE: And he continued working. You had a younger brother who would have been what age when your mother died?

ASHE: My brother was not a year old when my mother died.

CLARE: What kind of relationship did you have with him? Your brother.

ASHE: Well, I thought it was a normal older brother/younger brother relationship until I went to St Louis to finish my senior year in high school, when I was seventeen, and there we split up a little bit. But now that we're both well into adulthood we are, you know, renewing and nurturing our relationship. But it's quite different. I mean, he and I are very different. We're both driven, quite disciplined. He's a marine captain, so the essence of discipline, but our outlooks on life are not the same and our interests are not necessarily the same. But we're both driven. My father is the same way; we are achievers, no question about that, and also quite self-sufficient and self-reliant. That is, we're not the kind who'll want to naturally rely on somebody else to do something for us.

CLARE: Would you rely on anyone? Who would be someone without whom you mightn't survive? Is there such a person?

ASHE: Now after seven years and all that we've been through in seven years, without my wife it would be difficult. I can do it only because I don't think anything's impossible. But it would be difficult only because I've come to depend on her for certain things and those things are in areas where she has first-hand experience. Her father had a very serious heart attack in 1974, two years before we met, and she's gone through a heart attack with me and two heart operations.

CLARE: Have you children?

ASHE: No.

CLARE: Is that because of your medical history?

ASHE: Not completely. We're trying, it's just not always as easy as people think. You know aunts and uncles are always saying, you know, 'Well, when are we going to see some little ones running around,' and, you know, it's very difficult to say, 'Look, we want children just as badly as everybody else, but sometimes it just doesn't work.' The point I'm making is that everybody assumes that there's nothing the matter at all, ever.

CLARE: I asked merely because there's been a suggestion that it was related to the very heavy family loading on both sides of the Ashe family of cardiovascular disease.

ASHE: That's a consideration. As bad as my problem has been evidently, it's worse on my wife's side. Her brother, her older brother, died of a heart attack just a year ago, at thirty-nine. The heart disease problem is monumental in both of our families. When you take them together, it's staggering.

CLARE: How does that affect your perception of life? Is that something that has changed you? Is that one of those events that you mentioned?

ASHE: On, sure. That is an example of such an event. Of course that's something that would affect anybody's outlook, not just somebody like myself.

CLARE: But hitting you, as it did, in your thirties?

ASHE: Yes, that throws you for a loop because most people think that that should happen to people when they're in their sixties or seventies, where it's a normal time for it to happen. But you learn a bit about yourself, you rebound from it and you go on. For me, I guess it just makes you live a bit more for today than tomorrow. Long range planning for me is next month.

CLARE: Yes. What I missed somewhere in your account was

what I suppose I feel I would feel myself were it to happen to me, because we're around the same age, and that is this: there you were, riding very high in your career and you were a highly respected player and you had several years ahead of you still. Now what I missed, what may have been there, was a sense of anger, irrational maybe but that doesn't matter because I'm not talking about rationality for a minute, but just the anger when something like this strikes you on a court in Manhattan out of the blue and your life is changed.

ASHE: Yes, that anger is not unique, it happens to anybody who has such a thing happen to them at that age, which is not normal.

CLARE: It was there then?

ASHE: No, no, I wouldn't really call it anger. If you are black and born in the south before the mid fifties you get used to being knocked over the head with something, figuratively speaking or literally. You learn to evade certain situations or you learn to avoid them. You have to or else you wind up in jail or you'll be killed or you'll have a nervous breakdown. Life's very difficult for someone born black in the south before the fifties.

CLARE: Some of my more speculative colleagues sometimes tie bottled-up emotions with cardiovascular diseases.

ASHE: Oh, I firmly believe that they're correct, yes, absolutely. I mean that's just my subjective belief, yes.

CLARE: Well, making it even more personal, because you're describing in a sense an upbringing, a background, an early environment where to survive you had to maintain over yourself a lot of control.

ASHE: You have to internalise things, yes.

CLARE: Where does it come out with you, other than in your cardiovascular system? Do you ever lose your cool?

ASHE: No, almost never. I think because I would be personally embarrassed if I did, whereas most other people do it. John McEnroe does it and he's not embarrassed at all, or so it seems. I would be embarrassed. I think I would be embarrassed now at my age because I've never done it before, and people would go, 'Gee, that's odd, he doesn't normally do that,' and secondly because in the beginning we thought such outbursts would reflect back on us as a race. Here in the US, you'd have people say, 'You see what you get when you give a few of them an opportunity to do this, that or the other, they foul it up, they transgress codes of etiquette,' or whatever. Of course that's not true now. If I were coming along now, if I were ten years old now, I would be much freer to be like John McEnroe.

CLARE: Well, given that you're prepared to say, 'Yes, there is a connection,' you feel there is a connection between the way you cope and what happens to you physically, then in terms of prevention, prophylaxis over the next thirty years of your life, the message would seem to be that somehow that kind of way of coping has to change.

ASHE: Yes, that's difficult. You sound like a psychiatrist now! No, you're absolutely right. That's commonsense. You're right, you figure that would be very difficult to do? I don't know, I don't know. I don't think you even know too many people who in their forties can change their personalities.

CLARE: I agree, it's exceedingly difficult. It's not often I get an opportunity to hear someone like you in a completely different field, we're talking about physical ill health, we're not talking about psychiatry, saying just quite how you do it. Do you, for example, consciously reflect on the temperament that you've got and alter it or do you phlegmatically shrug your shoulders and say, 'I am what I am'?

ASHE: I don't want to say, 'I am what I am,' because I think that's a cop out. That imposes limits on me which I don't want. I don't want to think that I'm not capable of changing. Because if I said that I would also have to accept John McEnroe's statement to me that, 'Gee, I'm, you know, I just can't do it,' and if I look him in the face and say, 'Yes, you can,' well if John can change, then so can I. I guess it gets back to what I said about how I think others would see me if I did change.

CLARE: And that's still a factor?

ASHE: Oh, that's a factor with everyone, not just me. You see that with people who, for instance, have plastic surgery. You know they're more concerned with what other people think, other than what they think themselves when they look in the mirror just after the plastic surgery, to make themselves look better or just to change themselves.

CLARE: When you played and there was this notion of how you see yourself, how you'd wish others to see you, how they see you, it was inevitably tied in the late sixties, early seventies with the fact that you were black?

ASHE: Yes, that's always rock bottom, a huge part of it, because there are so many stereotypes about black athletes. There are stereotypes about athletes in general and even more about black athletes and that rankles. It rankles when I hear it. It rankles when I see evidences of it, as I do sometimes. Part of my life is a serious attempt on my part not to be in that lump but at the same time try to be someone whom other black athletes can point to and say, 'Look, that's ideally the way things should be done.'

CLARE: I wondered whether the kind of perception of the black athlete that you described, whether you encountered it at a place like Wimbledon?

ASHE: Oh, institutionally yes, not individually at all. I'm now a member of Wimbledon and I have never had any member of the staff or the officials ever treat me with anything but the utmost kindness. I don't think that was because I was Arthur Ashe. I've seen the way they treated other non-whites, other non-wasps so to speak, so in one sense Wimbledon represents institutionalised racial superiority only because it is a British tradition, and Britain I think, thinks of itself as God's gift to Western civilisation, along with a few Germans. But in actuality, Wimbledon as a tennis tournament tries to go the other way. In fact Wimbledon was the only event which for a long time, in its Junior Event for instance, admitted contestants solely on the basis of where they came from. They were more interested in a world-wide representation of players than they were in who the best players were. And so in that sense it epitomised again Britain's sense of fair play, something we, we don't have enough of over here in the US all the time.

CLARE: You've always reflected on yourself as a black in the United States and then in the world. You've had many things to say about, say, a country like South Africa. You were very influenced by Martin Luther King and Robert Kennedy and indeed by their deaths. I sense in you someone who could quite easily make the step into actual political life?

ASHE: No. I've thought about it. I've sort of been a leader of sorts all my life in the sense that I was always a part of student government in school, in the tennis organisations, the early ones, the antecedents to the Players Association, yes, I was always involved. I thought I might run for Congress or the Senate here in the US at some time but no, my heart condition, again, one of these critical junctures in my life, that's ruled that out completely.

CLARE: But it would have been something you considered? You did travel to South Africa several times.

ASHE: Yes, I've been there several times.

CLARE: When you were in South Africa, what kind of identity were you conscious of?

ASHE: That's a very interesting question because the second year that I went, a representative of the coloured section of South Africa said to me, 'Why don't you come over to our side of town, you're one of us, you spend too much time with the Africans.' Of all the statements I've heard in my time in South Africa for me personally that was the most telling statement, because a coloured South African saw me as being one of him, one of his group, whereas I identified most closely with the Africans.

CLARE: Do you remember what he said in relation to it? Was it merely a question of the shade of your colour?

ASHE: Well, down there a lot has to do with whether or not you know you have any white blood in you and down there coloureds obviously are the offspring of the unions, almost all of them illicit, between the Boers a long time ago and the Hottentots and so there are quite a few coloureds that live in South Africa, most in Cape Town. But it's just that he literally has been brain-washed into thinking that he's different. He also has been brain-washed into thinking that he is superior to the African, and possibly on a par with the Asian, but inferior to the white South African, and so he had bought this line, hook, line and sinker. And of course here in the US that, until, I would say, the sixties, socially was an unwritten rule here even in Black America. There are a lot of Black organisations wherein membership was open to blacks only but you had to be light-skinned, and your hair had to be a certain degree of straightness or else you would just not get in and that is still true today in a lot of places.

CLARE: In the United States?

ASHE: Oh, absolutely, especially if you saw, for instance, organisations whose members have been there for, let's say, twenty-five or thirty years. You would see, in a certain age range, the women looking pretty much the same, they would be fair-skinned blacks. If you were dark-skinned you just could not get in. And that's still true by and large today, in general, but much, much less so, no question about it.

CLARE: To an outsider, every American seems to have a duel citizenship, the Irish American, Polish American, German American, Italian American . . .

ASHE: You sound like *Moscow on the Hudson*, that movie!

CLARE: Quite, and in the sixties the American black appeared to find his second identity. I noticed in your book, I think it was your book, that you'd traced your family back to a slave landing in 1735 – HMS *Doddington*, I think it was. They were African slaves clearly. Now what impact did that have on you?

ASHE: Monstrous impact, yes, monstrous. Just as if, for no other reason than Prince Charles can trace his lineage back to however far he can trace it back, every English schoolboy and schoolgirl learns about it. Wouldn't it be wonderful, and wouldn't it make you a bit more secure, knowing where you came from and knowing what their achievements were? And we blacks just could not do that. We are, you know, just a hundred and twenty-one years out of slavery, and we haven't by any means gotten over it, I mean, not even close to getting over it yet. Well, you're talking about no more than five, six generations. We still, you know, many of us have the incorrect mentality for the 1980s.

CLARE: When you say an incorrect attitude, can you give me an example of what you mean?

ASHE: Incorrect, I mean, factually. I'm doing this book on the history of black American athletes which will be out in about a year and since I'm setting it in historical perspectives and I'm reading about racial attitudes in the late nineteenth century, early twentieth century, there is no question that very learned men at the Ivy League Schools, at Cambridge and Oxford, all thought that certain sorts of men, or races, or types, or cultures, were superior to others, maybe in technological terms or whatever. But certainly the ease with which the British Empire imposed its will over so many places – you know the adage that 'the sun never sets on a British flag' – had to lead people to think that, 'Hey, we have done this so it must be divinely ordained that we tell the rest of the world what to do.' There are still some people who think like that.

CLARE: And conversely within your own racial grouping, within the black consciousness in the United States, equally the irrational remnants of a sense of inferiority persist?

ASHE: Yes, absolutely, and the inferiority is unwittingly and sort of osmotically learned that the darker you are the more inferior you are, yes.

CLARE: And hence this point you made about the status related to the shade of the skin?

ASHE: Still very much an inhouse subject of discussion. You don't hear it discussed much between or among blacks and whites but within our own confines of our own group it's talked about a lot.

CLARE: In your book you mention the excitement of your first date with a white girl at UCLA. What was that like?

ASHE: Well, because, again, being a black southerner it was taboo. But also it was, I think, looking back on it now, a natural curiosity for anyone who is black, especially when you have been taught, and your ancestors even during and after slavery were taught, that the white woman was untouchable. In the south, you see, the white woman is put on a pedestal, much more so than in the north and she is made to feel that she's a queen and something that's just not to be defiled and not to have anything to do with lesser beings. And so you have a natural curiosity about white women. Every southern black man does. To a lesser extent I think every southern black woman has a curiosity about white men. But in California which is much more liberal, although not 180° different, nobody even bothers anymore about inter-racial marriages except black women. Black women, even educated black women, still hate it. By and large they don't like it at all.

CLARE: Black men marrying white women?

ASHE: Yes, and dating them because you see here in America now educated black women have a great deal of difficulty finding mates that they would like to spend the rest of their life with. It is very difficult. In fact the figures are that if you have a college degree, by the time you are thirty you'll be divorced with one child. Those chances are about six in ten. If you have a Masters degree and you are a black female, the chances are seven in ten that when you are thirty you won't be married at all. If you are looking for a black mate there just aren't enough black men that these super-educated black women can find to look up to, in a conventional sense. So black women, even educated ones, highly educated, supposedly very rational ones, hate it if you marry outside the race, especially if you yourself are black and educated. And obviously the paradox is that the black male who is very well educated, let's say if he had a Phd or Masters, feels even freer to pick whomever he likes as a partner. You feel less free the further down you go on the educational attainment scale.

CLARE: Do you go much to the south, because you're from the south?

ASHE: Sure, yes, but you never leave the south. If you were born in the south that's where you were born, no matter where you go you're always southern. Even black southerners want to defend the south. Here in America northerners have looked upon southerners as being backwards. Because the weather is so much warmer and the pace is so much slower, northerners think southerners are lazy and indolent and up to no good, shiftless etc, and black southerners dislike that as much as white southerners. Southern accents, for instance, are just no-nos, if you want to get a good job. For instance, if you go to a southern city now, Alabama, or Mobile or Montgomery or Atlanta or Mississippi, you turn on any radio station, any powerful radio station, say, at 50,000 watts, or around that, the accent will be distinctly northern. You don't put a local who has a local southern drawl on a very important radio station or TV station in the south.

CLARE: Has your accent changed?

ASHE: My accent changed, yes. I no longer sound the way I sounded when I was a kid. But if I go home and stay three or four days I can sort of unwittingly lapse back. I don't lapse back into it as far as word selection, but the accent.

CLARE: The impression I obtained from reading about you, Arthur, was that you had given the subject of death a great deal of thought. Even when you were quite young you give an account of a personal fascination with death, visiting cemeteries. A visit to the morgue I think you once described.

ASHE: It's not an obsession, and I certainly want to die, or rather I want to live, as long as I can, and I don't think that slip was a Freudian slip either. (*Laugh.*) I've even had, upon occasion, in a lighter vein, some palm readers read my palm and say, 'Oh, you've got a long life-line here, you're going to live a long time,' and I say, 'Yippee.' I mean I want to live as long as the next person. But if you've had a heart attack in your thirties and you've had two heart operations and you have studied, as a layman, heart disease, what causes it and what its mortality complications are and so forth, then I know what's going on inside of me and so I don't think I will live to the maximum. But how concerned and how obsessed I am about it, it's not debilitating at all. But I do keep my will up to date and I've even gone so far as to write out instructions about what's to be done if I do die, because I don't want people having to fight about, no that's a strong word, discuss what I want done with me, so it's all written down. Now I don't think that means I am obsessed psychotically or neurotically with death. But the boyishness in me, the boy in me, the little boy in me, wonders if I will see my mother again, if I die, that makes the spectre of dying more palatable. Maybe I will in some form see her again – wanting to see her again is very powerful, but I'm not willing to die prematurely to do it. It's just that that's another way of sort of lessening its negative impact so to speak.

CLARE: Was that one of the factors that accounted for your interest in death before you ever had your coronaries?

ASHE: No, I mean it crossed my mind but no, it didn't account for it. No question about it, my heart attack made my mortality something that I would put on the front burner so to speak.

CLARE: Has it affected your sense of priorities?

ASHE: Yes. It makes today more important than tomorrow or the day after.

CLARE: You exude a certain kind of acceptance, not stoicism so much as easiness. Are you a man who could get, did get, does get occasionally profoundly gloomy?

ASHE: No, I never get depressed, almost never. One of the reasons is because, again going back to the biographies I've read, I've always tried to have something, a central focus in my life, other than family I mean. Right now it's this book on the black American athlete that I'm writing, that's something I want to see get done, and I don't have time to get gloomy.

CLARE: So setbacks, either in tennis when you were an active player, losing something, throwing it away, a blunder, or the disease, being stricken down . . .?

ASHE: That's all normal. Those are things that happened to countless people in the past and I'm just another one. I've always tried to structure my life so that if any one part didn't work then I had something else to fall back on that would make life worthwhile without the missing part. So I had my heart attack, thank God if I'm going to have it, at thirty-six, towards the end of my career. Thirty-six is not a bad age, tennis-wise, to have a heart attack if you're going to have one, because your best is behind you. And so that even makes the decision to retire easy. You retire, and then you go on to some other things that you've thought about doing with your life while you were playing. Now I always liked writing and so now I'm doing a lot of writing.

CLARE: Yes. Just one last question. If, or should I say when, you meet your mother what would you say? What would you ask?

ASHE: I don't think I would say anything, I'd probably just let her hold me for a while, for a long time. Yes, that's because I can't recall that ever having happened.

Dame Janet Baker

I am often asked why people consent to being interviewed. Usually the questioner promptly advances an answer before I can formulate one myself. People consent, I am assured, because they are narcissistic, they enjoy talking about themselves. Well, that is true. To varying extents we all enjoy talking about ourselves. In a world of increasing complexity almost the only thing any of us can still claim to have substantial competence about and knowledge of is ourselves. We should not be too surprised that given half a chance to talk about ourselves so many of us readily grab it. Then again, it is suggested that people agree to interviews because they are flattered to be asked. It boosts their morale and reassures them that they are still important. I do recall Arnold Wesker very frankly acknowledging that one of his motives for accepting my invitation was indeed to help keep his name in the public eye. Some admit to curiosity about the experience – a way of meeting a psychiatrist without having to go through the dreary business of developing symptoms! And some, like Dame Janet Baker, accept the invitation because it enables them to put the record straight. Rather as an autobiography allows a person to tell it his or her way, unadorned by other perspectives and unedited by other hands, so this interview provides the subject with a greater opportunity to put his or her account of life, motives, drives and experiences without fear of misrepresentation. That indeed is a strength of the interview. It is of course also its weakness. No other voice is heard. Fathers, mothers, siblings, spouses, lovers are described, praised, condemned, dismissed, beatified with no corresponding third party evidence to support or challenge this version of the truth.

At the heart of Dame Janet Baker's interview is a curious revelation – that the singer from time to time, perhaps all the time, sees herself as separate from her very remarkable voice. With precious little prompting from me, she proceeded to describe her voice as 'the most crushing responsibility'. Where did such a perception originate? Ambition is usually although not invariably fuelled by a mentor, a parent, a teacher, an older sibling. She discounted them all. No, she was to insist, she herself was the source of this very personal vision.

I was then and I remain now doubtful. There is another possibility, one for which Janet Baker herself provides intriguing evidence. As a small girl she sang in a church choir with Peter, a brother four years her senior. Peter, if her mother is to be believed, had a truly superb voice. But Peter was to die tragically of rheumatic heart disease at the tender age of fourteen. And what then does her mother do? She announces to the bewildered Janet that she is to bear Peter's gift, his beautiful voice. So in a very particular sense Janet Baker's truly marvellous voice is not her own, is not an intrinsic part of herself but is a voice apart, is someone else's. It is her brother's. But she now assumes absolute responsibility for its cultivation, development, triumph. She herself declares at one point in the interview that her voice has a 'divine' purpose. Split from her and separate, it embodies perfection, it demands worship. She is a vessel 'carrying a divine attribute'. It is a cross to be carried for the spiritual enrichment of others. Were she to neglect it, impair it in any way she would enter a state of sin. It is hardly surprising in the circumstances that she uses terms like 'crushing burden', 'crushing load'.

Years later her mother dies and Janet starts to dream about her and their relationship. There is a recurrent theme, a predictable and common enough one, a dream of sibling rivalry. Peter is the preferred child. His death was indeed shattering. Janet Baker watched him die peacefully but as she described in her autobiography *Full Circle* published in 1984 'the grief in our house was like a mountain pressing down upon me. What this death did to me I shall never know. It certainly did something.' (The memory of her brother's death is triggered in her book by a news report of the death of little boys in a Beaconsfield train crash on 11 December 1981. 'I know what the parents of these small boys are going through at the present moment; snow, ice, a howling wind blowing and

Christmas, the feast of children, looming up ahead; for these families, Christmas will never be the same again.' For her parents thus it proved. 'My parents,' she observed elsewhere, 'never got over losing their son. They were wounded people.'

People who lose a child never get over it. They struggle to cope in various ways, some of which can have unexpected and unintended consequences for those children who remain. J. M. Barrie's mother's reaction to the death of his older brother, for example, was so extreme, so catastrophic that she utterly withdrew from the mute, bewildered, pathetic James leaving him to grieve in perplexity outside her bedroom door listening to her ceaseless sobbing. Janet Baker's mother does not appear to have reacted in such a pathological way. Indeed, their relationship remained intense and strong until her mother's death. But there is nonetheless in Janet Baker some residue of competition with the memory of her dead brother, of a striving for unqualified love, a demand for recognition that has not so much to do with a superb voice as a small girl troubled by the fact that her stricken mother has other matters on her mind.

How much too of the religious language which she employs to describe her talent and professional career reflects a deep-seated, perhaps unconscious belief that her brother's death has been a sacrifice made to enable her to live, prosper, succeed, fulfil her own destiny? Throughout her reflections on her life and art threads a profound melancholy, a nagging doubt of the ultimate worth of her endeavour, the price paid in blood and sweat. 'If someone asked me if my career has been "worth it",' she wrote in her autobiography, 'in other words worth the sacrifices made by me and members of my family, worth the separations, the agony of performing, of trying to keep perfectly fit, the undying battle against nerves, the strains and pitfalls of being a public figure, my honest answer would have to be "No" . . . The moments when the musical rewards have equalled the price one has to pay for them have been few.'

The problem with a brief interview, for that is all such an interview can hope to be, is that there is only limited time to open up issues, not develop them. I recall leaving the very first interview I ever did in *In the Psychiatrist's Chair* (with Glenda

Jackson), my mind full of her words and the questions I would put to her at our next 'session' — only to remember that of course there would not be a next session, that this was it. So I remain intrigued by the seeming contradictions in Janet Baker's demand to be normal, treated as normal, regarded as ordinary, in no way extraordinary and her irritability with members of her family when they do treat her in precisely that way — her example of her family's failure to recognise the impact of the common cold on her voice being a case in point. There is a thin line between egotism and professional concern, between narcissism and a performer's dedication to the cultivation of talent but it is a line that is damnably difficult to draw. Janet Baker herself acknowledges the dilemma in her discussion about having children. 'I didn't think it was right to put my music second,' she declares, 'neither did I think it was right to put my children second, which is why I made the decision not to have any.' Where she appears to draw this thin line is between herself and her voice; she is a very ordinary woman, once second in her mother's affections to a very remarkable brother who died in a state of perfection, now married to an understanding, supportive man; her voice is divine, spiritual, of another world. When Janet Baker puts herself first it is not for her sake but for her voice. Here she articulates the artist's dilemma and demand. It leaves those ordinary mortals around her with a simple choice — acknowledge the demands of her divine attribute or leave her be.

A man articulating this dilemma and concluding that his profession, talent, skill came first would excite little comment. Who amongst us thinks the less of a surgeon who puts his vocation before his domestic responsibilities, a painter his canvas before his wife? But Janet Baker coolly discussing the choice between child and voice comes face to face with the accusation of selfishness. Leaving aside that moral judgement, consider again the significance this 'voice' assumes. It transcends art and acquires a religious significance. One critic of this modern identification of art with religion, Jacques Barzun, has observed that there is a view that suggests that the artist, like the worshipper, 'gives himself over to an experience so very different from those of the ordinary self that he deems it loftier, truer, more lasting.'[1] By its nature art is seen to express the deepest and the best in man. Art liberates. Art transcends. Janet Baker, expounding a profoundly religious view of her splendid voice, is actually describing her life as a singer as a form of religious vocation, not willingly chosen but visited upon her and born with stoic forebearance.

Her views on men, women and sexuality only serve to raise additional questions though again there is more than a suggestion that sexuality like everything else has to be subordinated to her calling. But sexuality, particularly male sexuality, is difficult to tame. Janet Baker's view of herself and her voice recalls Schiller's division of mankind into the alienated, unhappy, self-conscious man, always examining motives and impulses and questioning his purpose and worth, and the artist, simple, childlike, natural, spontaneous and free. Where one proceeds with anxious, deliberate caution, the other acts by feeling and inspiration. The artist, in this model, Barzun suggests, 'is inspired by self-belief, which gives him power, a magnetic attraction and control over others, like a saint or a great leader of men.'

Once a therapist to whom she went after her mother died and who helped her learn to meditate told her that her gift had been given to her for her own enjoyment as well as for other people's. She had never thought of that before. It helped her cope with the terrible anxiety she experienced before going on stage to perform. But she has not totally convinced herself of its truth. How, for example, does she describe the moment of supreme achievement, of adulation, of acclamation at the end of a triumphant concert at one of the great cathedrals of her art, say Carnegie Hall? Yes of course the applause is for her but only in the most superficial of senses. More accurately, it is for her gift, that divinely inspired voice. She the vessel is 'just like a fallible human being'. It does not appear false modesty merely

[1] *The Use and Abuse of Art*, Jacques Barzun, Princeton University Press, Princeton, 1975.

a recognition of the dilemma faced by any ordinary human being graced and burdened by a spark of genius.

CLARE: Dame Janet Baker was born in Hatfield, near Doncaster on 21 August 1933. Her father was an electrical engineer, her mother a full-time housewife and she had one brother, Peter, who died of heart disease aged 14 when she herself was 10 years old. After singing in local choirs she began studying under Helene Ysep in 1953, and in 1956 won second prize in the Kathleen Ferrier Award and that summer, she joined the Glyndebourne Chorus and began what was to prove to be an outstanding professional career in opera, in concert and in the recording studio. In 1976 she was awarded the D.B.E.

CLARE: Janet Baker, you describe yourself as a private person, why do you consent to talk about yourself?

BAKER: Because my words are mine. They aren't put into my mouth, or written down in an angled way or in a way that is untrue. I think if somebody hears you speak they know that it's coming from you, it's not being manipulated in any way.

CLARE: In contrast to what, then?

BAKER: Well, newspapers.

CLARE: Have you over the years been someone who has suffered that kind of misrepresentation?

BAKER: I think every public person, having given an interview, would open a newspaper or a magazine and think, 'Well, was it really like that?', and then the answer is – no it wasn't really like that. You can't recognise yourself through most interviews and the thing that rather disturbs me about journalism is that these days it's considered permissible to put in quotation marks sentences that you know you have never spoken, and that is really very dangerously misrepresentation I think.

CLARE: Yes. Yes.

BAKER: It frightens all of us.

CLARE: And is there a side of you, an aspect of you which you feel has been profoundly misrepresented in a consistent way?

BAKER: No, I can't say that with all honesty. I would say that I'm finding out that people in my profession have a very different picture of me from the one I have of myself and the one I think that they have.

CLARE: That's interesting. What sort of picture?

BAKER: I'll tell you something very funny that happened about two weeks ago. I was adjudicating a prize at the Royal Academy of Music. I went there fairly early morning on the train, because it's hopeless bringing the car in at that time of day, and when I got to the front door I saw a huge Rolls Royce parked with two wheels on the pavement bang in front of the entrance so that it was very difficult to get in or out. And I thought 'Gosh, what a selfish thing, whoever owns that car, to park it so blatantly and so blatantly in an inconvenient place.' Well, as the morning went on I kept getting reports from people coming into the room saying 'Everybody thinks that's your car out there, everybody thinks it's your car. Is it your car?' And of course it was not my car. I don't have a Rolls Royce. I wouldn't park it there inconveniencing everybody so blatantly and so arrogantly, but that's what they think I would do. That's how they think a successful person behaves and it pains me to think that that is the picture people have of somebody like me.

CLARE: Yes. You've actually answered the question about being interviewed quite differently from almost everybody else I've asked. So that's why I'm sticking with it for a second. Has anybody ever suggested that there was a sort of callous side to you, that there was a hidden life that you were involved in, in some strange way, quite different from your public and personal appearance?

BAKER: You mean the scandal. Oh yes. Every so often stories filter back to us about the latest extraordinary thing that I am supposed to have done. It's not easy having lies spread about one, but it happens to the Queen, so it can happen to everybody else I suppose. It's an annoyance and it really is an interesting phenomena because it also teaches one, if you survive it, a very useful way of looking at oneself. I think perhaps it's important for people in public life at some point to feel stripped, and this is what this process does. The stupidity, the gossip, the lies, strip you of a false picture probably you have of yourself.

CLARE: How much of that lay behind your decision to publish *Full Circle*?

BAKER: Well, quite a lot of it because when the final year of my operatic life came around – things seem to slot into patterns in my life. Probably this happens to a lot of people, but I certainly noticed this. My life, in some extraordinary way, if I allow it intuitively and don't say 'Well, I'm going to do this, that and the other,' plans itself in the most remarkable way. This happened to my last year in opera. It happened with the decision to write about the last year in opera, and I thought when I embarked on this diary that once I'd done it, and said what I wanted to say, my life really wasn't of any material use to anybody else, because it's been done by me, and therefore they might leave me alone.

CLARE: And did they?

BAKER: Yes.

CLARE: One of the most moving recollections in that book occurs – I think it's in December of 1980–1. It's the day that there's a train crash in Beaconsfield and some children were killed and you then write as if it's yesterday about the death of your brother, Peter.

BAKER: Yes. I think that devastating experience must have scarred me in ways I'm not even aware of now. I'm sure it did.

CLARE: Just looking at that for a second. He was the older brother, there were two of you, and with his death you became the only child.

BAKER: Yes.

CLARE: Looking at that in terms of the relationship with your parents, what changed?

BAKER: I think I assumed a responsibility for them, for their happiness, which was too great a burden for me to bear. I've tried to be a good daughter, I think perhaps I've tried to be too good a daughter, if one can say that, I really do. I don't regret it, I don't regret anything that's happened to me in my whole life, but I can see that that traumatic experience did something to me which I've had to pay for.

CLARE: Is it related, do you think, to the other thing that you have written about on a number of occasions, and that is the fact that for much of your life you had a tendency to see your talent as something other people enjoyed. You had difficulty taking pleasure in life and in things, and particularly your voice, your talent?

BAKER: Yes. I think it's bound up with fear. Probably the two things are — interestingly enough I've never thought about it quite like that — a connecting, this feeling of responsibility. I certainly have felt that my voice has been the most crushing responsibility and part of my agony as a performer has been to cope with this sense of inadequacy while being asked to fulfil a destiny which I didn't feel — not incapable of, but worthy of, let's say.

CLARE: Worthy of?

BAKER: That changed of course, it changed.

CLARE: These values of things like worthy, the crushing responsibility — you speak in these terms, they would have been part of the value structure of the family, this north of England family?

BAKER: Yes, I suppose so.

CLARE: Your father comes across as a man who was relatively easy about your talent. Am I wrong about that?

BAKER: No, I don't think you are wrong. He doesn't make any demands now. He's still alive at 83. He takes it all very — quite lightly actually, I don't mean to say that he doesn't realise what I've achieved, not that at all, but I don't think it would have bothered him at all whether I'd been famous or not. I don't think it would my mother either. I think they wanted to see me successful, but fame wasn't something they understood or expected from me.

CLARE: But who was the first crucial influential person who seemed to regard this voice with awe, who, in other words, made you? Because you talk of it, as sometimes — as if it's something else, outside you.

BAKER: Me. Me.

CLARE: It was you.

BAKER: Yes. It was me. I felt it in my teens when I left home. I was very unhappy when I left home. I felt very homesick and very lost without my roots, and I had a pretty hard time of it as a student here . . .

CLARE: In London?

BAKER: Yes. But I couldn't run away from that. I felt very much that my voice was a — something, nothing to do with me, that it had been given to me at birth and it was a duty to make the most of it if I possibly could.

CLARE: You were the sort of vessel.

BAKER: Yes.

CLARE: Carrying precious cargo.

BAKER: That's right.

CLARE: What sort of student were you. I mean, late adolescence, were you gawky, did you feel physically attractive?

BAKER: Very boring, I think, very boring.

CLARE: Did you have boyfriends?

BAKER: Not at — no, I didn't have time really. I was working and working very hard to try and keep body and soul together and my parents were helping with my music lessons so I felt again a sense of responsibility, there was no time really for much of a social life. I'd have liked one, but . . .

CLARE: Yes, what kind of a person were you, were you shy? You say private, were you shy?

BAKER: Yes, I think so yes, I think so. I think so, I would say that still about myself. I am a very shy person.

CLARE: Were you the sort of girl who'd prefer not to be asked questions in public?

BAKER: No, no. My brother always used to think I was a frightful show-off, but that was because I had this inner feeling of confidence about being destined for something, and therefore that confidence I had as a little girl probably looked like brashness. It probably does as an adult, and people who know me might say, listening to this 'Oh gosh, she's not shy, she's anything but shy.' In a way that is true. In a way there is a deeply private and personal part of me which finds performing a great intrusion into my inner life, but nevertheless that's something I have to give.

CLARE: This sense of responsibility, we started to discuss this in terms of the effect of the death of your brother. Around what time did you realise you had a voice?

BAKER: Very difficult to answer that, because I've always sung, I don't know how well I sung, but I'd always sung and from about nine years old when I was in the church choir with my brother – we were both in the church choir – I was aware of having authority. When I opened my mouth I felt, and still feel, as whole as I do at any time. My feeling of oneness, my feeling of total reality is when I open my mouth and make music and that I suppose was true at nine years old. I had this feeling of 'I know how this is to be done, I know I'm right.'

CLARE: So even before Peter's death you knew you had a gift.

BAKER: Yes. Yes. And my mother made a very strange remark after he died, because he had a very good voice too, and when he died she said to me 'Oh, you've been given Peter's gift', and I bridled at that, I would not entertain that at all. I said, 'No, it's nothing to do with my brother, this is my gift, it's nothing at all to do with him, this is mine', as though she was trying to allay him on to me. I wouldn't have that even at that early age.

CLARE: Have you felt responsibility of that kind?

BAKER: Since my mother's death ten years ago I have had many dreams about her and about our relationship. I used to get dreams of being little, with my brother still alive, and my mother, the three of us, and in my dreams I used to be saying to her, 'I know you love him better than you do me, but don't worry about it, it doesn't matter,' and I would wake . . . Because I've always said, I've always thought and always said that my mother was very, very fair with both of us. He was an invalid, and totally different in looks and character from me. I realised because he was sick that she had to give him something different, but I didn't feel as a child that I was being pushed out. But in the dreams that I had, much, much later, something seemed to be telling me that as a little child I might have resented the energy and the time that they had together, but I wasn't aware of it. I was aware of it in adult life. I seemed to be aware that maybe she did love him better than me, maybe in some strange way it would have been better if I'd died instead. She never, she would never ever have admitted that, and this is something that is my problem, not theirs. It wasn't the problem. It's just something that I've been trying to iron out in adult life that perhaps, perhaps she did love him best, and if she did, well then I have to accept that.

CLARE: You certainly wrote agonizingly about the impact on her of his death.

BAKER: Oh, yes. Yes.

CLARE: You saw very tangibly. In watching someone's reaction to someone else's death you see the intensity of a love.

BAKER: Oh, yes, yes you do. She never recovered from it. I don't think so, until she was an old lady, she never recovered from it.

CLARE: In what way?

BAKER: She couldn't really speak about him without tremendous distress and longing and it was obviously like an open bleeding wound. Probably for my father too. I'm not saying that he didn't feel exactly the same way, but men show these things differently. I think it wounded them both irretrievably, but for my mother the wound was always open.

CLARE: One of the roles that you're famous for is Alceste, and you wrote there about this extraordinary role where the central figure loses husband and children, describing how you summon up that kind of understanding. You talked of drawing on your pool of loss, and you didn't say what loss it was, but I assumed it was that one.

BAKER: Yes, yes, absolutely, and the loss of my mother. I mean she was a wonderful mother to me, and although I have been trying to become a separate person from her in the years since she died, nevertheless I am bound to my mother, to her memory and to what she did for me, and – I feel her loss terribly now.

CLARE: Really. Was she a powerful figure?

BAKER: Very powerful. Very powerful. Very gifted, totally thwarted in her intelligence and in her artistic gift and her philosophy on life. We could talk in a most amazing way about everything and in a way again there is that sense of responsibility. I had everything that was denied her in the end.

CLARE: Did she envy you?

BAKER: I think probably she would have done, yes, I think perhaps she did.

CLARE: Was that what you meant when you wrote about a certain conflict between, I suppose, you the performer, the artist, and this background? In a sense there was a distance opened up.

BAKER: I don't think there was a distance because I wouldn't allow that to happen.

CLARE: You were conscious of it?

BAKER: Yes I was. I walk in two worlds and I think I'm not the only performer who has discovered this, that the roots are quite a long way away from the actual life you find yourself in as a professional person, and I think it's very, very dangerous to discard them.

CLARE: Was it a conflict?

BAKER: I just longed for family life in general to understand what I was going through in terms of – of what was being taken from me by my work, and yet I had to deny myself as a performer, in order to try and appear normal. Everybody wants me to be ordinary and normal in the normal side of my life and that was as great an act for me as it was to be on the stage.

CLARE: They would have been quick to spot any tendency of Janet Baker to be extraordinary.

BAKER: Yes, that's not allowed.

CLARE: Can you give an example of what you would have liked to have been with them, but just couldn't.

BAKER: Well, I would have liked people to understand a very

simple thing, like how tragic the common cold can be for a singer. Some members of my family were, and are still, extremely conscientious about coming near me with a streaming cold. Other members of the family, although we tried to explain it time after time, seemed to discount the fact that to come near me with a streaming cold at the start of an opera run, or at any time, was scandalous, but you know, it never did get through. It's a very basic, seemingly trivial thing, but not a trivial thing to me. Now that kind of respect or care, they don't, they don't understand the kind of care a person like me has to have.

CLARE: Would this have been thoughtless, or do you think that there actually would have been a few feeling that this is Janet Baker having airs and graces – what's a common cold.

BAKER: Well, you see, if you tell somebody, ten or fifteen times, the common cold is a tragedy for me, and they still don't take any notice, what are you to think? I don't know.

CLARE: But occasionally you thought murderous thoughts.

BAKER: Yes.

CLARE: About this thing about the voice, did you ever hate it? Did you ever wish it would go away?

BAKER: Oh no. Never. But then, if you have a – I won't say it's a driving ambition, it wasn't a driving ambition, it was a driving force that I felt I was born to do this particular thing, and that it was a divine purpose, that's the thing. Oh, we always go back to this, that it wasn't an ego trip, it's never been that. My career, in the strict sense of the word, what has driven me, is this feeling that I've been given something and that that can't be ignored or run away from or denied in any way, either by me, or by anybody else. And that if it meant agony personally for me to fulfil this destiny, then too bad, I had to go through with it.

CLARE: A little like a religious vocation?

BAKER: Yes.

CLARE: Straining against it, but not yours to determine.

BAKER: Absolutely.

CLARE: How related is this idea that you have, this belief that you have about your voice, how related is it to the fact that you never had children?

BAKER: I don't think it's anything to do with that at all. I don't see how it could possibly be anything to do with that, because I felt this sense of calling and purpose and meaning since being a tiny little girl. What I was very conscious of was the fact that children would come first in my life, and that I didn't think that was right. I didn't think it was right to put my music second, neither did I think it was right to put children second, which is why I made the decision not to have any.

CLARE: You did. It was an absolute, definite decision?

BAKER: Absolutely, absolutely.

CLARE: It's the sort of decision that people do question you about.

BAKER: Oh, very much, yes. People think it's very selfish, and they did thirty years ago when my husband and I made it. The way I feel about children is to put children second would be a selfish thing to do. In my opinion. I could not be the kind of mother I would want to be with my mind and my physical body so engrossed in something else. But I've always made it so absolutely clear that while for some women that is not a conflict, it is for me. And I recognised it immediately. So, you know, one has a certain amount of energy and a certain amount to give, you can't go beyond that, and I knew that both my music and my children would have suffered and I couldn't bear that.

CLARE: Was it a difficult decision?

BAKER: No.

CLARE: No?

BAKER: Not in the least. Actually, physically, I would not have been able to have children, as it turned out.

CLARE: Because?

BAKER: Because of my physical equipment, which started going wrong when I was twenty-eight, and I was told by my gynaecologist at forty that it would have been absolutely not unheard of, but extremely unlikely. So even my body was backing up that decision.

CLARE: You've talked about the tremendous strain of pre-performance particularly. You talk of waking up and groaning, and that this is performance day, and so on. Do you feel when you're on that you are, so to speak, 'at home'?

BAKER: Now, yes. But it's taken me practically all my performing life to be able to say yes to that question. Until a very short time ago the whole problem of getting out there has been so enormous that I would think, 'God, I hope I'll never be born into this kind of life again. I hope I'll never be born as a performer again,' but not now, not now. I feel, I always did feel, more whole out there than any other time, more real, more myself, although going through all this agony. Now I feel, well, to have achieved what I now feel is the most extraordinary development I think any human being could ask for, because not only am I still able to perform well, but all these chains have fallen off. All these agonies, all this pain and all this struggle has gone and I am allowed to share in it and to be, in that moment of music-making, like the audience is. I can share in the whole process in a way that I never could before. That is the most indescribable privilege and joy. This is it. It's the element of joy which has entered into my life which wasn't there before, and it's − I can't tell you how grateful I am for that.

CLARE: There is in the heart of this quite an emphasis on you alone, aloneness.

BAKER: Yes.

CLARE: You have a very remarkable marriage. You married in your twenties someone from a very similar background, Keith, and he's been your companion through this journey, right through.

BAKER: Absolutely.

CLARE: Now, this must call for a very particular kind of marriage, in view of what you have said.

BAKER: Yes, I think my whole life calls for quite exceptional circumstances. Again, to me it's an absolute illustration of the kind of loving care which I've been aware of in my circumstances. All my circumstances have been making the kind of life I've lived possible − the care of my parents, their support of me, even though they didn't know much about music, but nevertheless they trusted it was going to be all right. The fact that I met a man who could not be more perfect for the kind of human being I needed. We fell in love very passionately and extraordinarily when we were young so that I didn't choose him for having this talent. I didn't say 'Oh this is going to be a good partner for me'. I married for the usual completely nonsensical reasons people usually get married for. But the fact remains that, in retrospect, again this person came for me who was so absolutely right in many, many different ways including his own attitude towards what I had to do. There's a great deal of unselfishness there. I suppose in a way I'm quite difficult to live with.

CLARE: In what way?

BAKER: Well, I'm moody. I have big mood swings and I have a lot of imagination, you know people, imaginative people are not easy and I'm not, I'm not an even keel. He is, he's a very balanced person – he's the counter-balance to me flying up into the stratosphere.

CLARE: Let me ask you something. Susan Hill, I think it was, she wrote of your book, that in it you were exposing yourself and all your deepest, most private reflections to public scrutiny. Now, in fact, in that book we've touched on some of the things – you certainly write of grief and sacrifice and loss, you write of very personal decisions like not having children. You write of religious belief which I know is very private to you and you, rightly in my view, object to people saying 'Are you religious?' and asking these profound questions in these crude ways. One of the things that isn't in the book very much is sexuality.

BAKER: True, yes. Quite true.

CLARE: And I supposed I wondered why, in a sense that a lot of other very personal things were.

BAKER: I used the word boring of myself when I was a student, and in a way I think I am boring as a woman. I don't feel attractive to the opposite sex. I don't want to be involved in all the to-ing and fro-ing of a flirtatious relationship with a man. I have a few good men friends, but I suppose part of my boringness is the fact that because I consider myself married my background means that I'm off limits, and therefore I don't want to go into the area where this is in jeopardy. It's as simple as that really, being brought up where I was, in the north of England, and how I was. A married woman is a married woman and that's how I think of myself. I am not available in any other way to a man, and I find it quite difficult, actually, to be friends with men in general because men, I have found, expect woman to react to their light-hearted conversation or suggestive conversation, I don't like suggestive conversation. I don't like a man telling me dirty stories, I hate it. I don't like a man looking down the front of my frock or anything – it makes me feel awkward, and in that sense I suppose I can't cope with masculinity in the way that a sophisticated woman should be able to.

CLARE: Do you find it easier to have that kind of close relationship with a woman?

BAKER: Well, because of my generation, talking about my background and the way I was brought up, it was all right to have girlfriends, but a boyfriend was a different thing. A girlfriend to me was OK but a boyfriend meant something else besides a friend, and I suppose I still feel that to a certain extent.

CLARE: Because of the nature of the singing that you have done over the years, the parts that you have played, some of them stir you to reflections. I notice that one of the things you reflect on is this conflict between Apollo and Dionysus, the conflict between rationality and control. You talk about the ideal being some kind of balance. Do you think you have that balance, or are you more Apollonian than Dionysian?

BAKER: Oh, I think I am, yes, but, this is what I am learning about, you see, the putting of my arms around darknesses, I think is a very, very important task for me. We all have this maze of difficulty to get through and I grew to understand that one of my major difficulties was thinking that this crushing load, this crushing burden which my music, my gift, had imposed upon me was of my own making. That not being able to accept my ego, my human bit as a paradox of light and dark made me judgemental and that I would go on to the platform and think my God, you know, it'll never be good enough, and, of course, it never was good enough. Of course it never could be because I wanted to be as a human being divine, I suppose. What an arrogance! I was thinking of myself as this sort of vessel carrying a divine attribute. OK the divine attribute had been put into a very human person a˙d at last I have been able to recognise that and think this is good, with all its faults and failings, this is how it is, this gift is in a human body and there's nothing I can do about that and I'm certainly not going to apologise for it any more, which is the load rolled away.

CLARE: And it happened when?

BAKER: About six years ago.

CLARE: Yes.

BAKER: Since then, on the platform when I now feel free to give of myself totally, when they're all in Carnegie Hall shouting and clapping and everybody saying, 'Oh darling, how marvellous,' I can absolutely truly say to you, that I stand on the platform and I think, 'Yes, OK, there you are, clapping who you think is me, fine, that's fine, but it isn't me.' This is something other that I am not responsible for, that I'm sharing in just like anybody else, but I don't have the responsibility for it. I can share it and it's there and I suppose it's a part of me in a sense, but I don't have to be crushingly perfect in order to sustain this gift. I'm sharing in it just like a fallible human being, and that I think's the most useful lesson I've learnt in all my life.

Ken Dodd

I interviewed Ken Dodd before the storm over tax and his difficulties with the Inland Revenue broke around his head. There is only a brief reference to the subject of money during the interview — based it has to be said on the fact that people who had spoken to me about Dodd before I met him had suggested that he had a tendency to be tight-fisted. There are hints, nothing more, of an anxiety about money, of being short of it, a suggestion of hoarding (denied — although admitted with regard to newspapers, magazines). Instead the interview, as often happens, tends to become focused on a couple of themes that recur throughout. In Ken Dodd's case they are his religious sense of some kind of purpose or destiny and his status as a loner, someone who lives alone, has never married and despite his stated interest in and desire for children has never had any.

Ken Dodd in the studio was not a relaxed man although he exuded a cheery bonhomie and was both genuine and amusing. Many comedians are not particularly funny away from the stage or cameras — one thinks of Tony Hancock, Frankie Howerd, Tommy Cooper — but Dodd was and from time to time would without much obvious effort reproduce the stream of puns, made-up words, incongruous images and corny jokes which are his trademark. He clearly wanted to formulate some kind of theory of comedy (perhaps he felt that it was what I was in search of) and made the usual suggestions, comedy as a return to childhood, as anarchic response to repression, as an adult version of the fundamentally human spirit of play.

The interview, like many, generated considerable correspondence. Some wondered why I had spent so much time exploring Dodd's bachelor status and attitudes to children and family life. It is a fair comment. In fact, it owes something to the fact that from the moment I raised these themes Ken Dodd used his considerable abilities to distract me. There is about him, and certainly about his comic turns, a marked element of control. Ken Dodd's monologues are not so much about communications with members of an audience, as he often argues, as about bludgeoning them into helpless, hysterical insensibility. The stream of words, the rapid changes of pace, topic and mood, all serve to render an audience powerless. Rightly or wrongly, Dodd's need to control intrigued me — hence the questions on hoarding, punctuality, the performance — and right away I sensed a battle within the studio for control of the subject matter, a battle I lost.

Ken Dodd talked fluently, rapidly, steadily in this interview. Confronted with areas of life that are difficult to control — love, sex, dependence — he would change gear, change the subject. Returning to them was a struggle and yes it does look as if it is I who has the fixations. So when I eventually do turn him back to the paradox of love of family, love of children, fond reminiscences of his own early childhood, he promptly and neatly observes, 'You've got a thing about this haven't you?'

Well, yes as a matter of fact I have. And it is a curiosity about the extent that we are or are not the products of our early years as so much of the conventional psychological wisdom insists. I don't think I get any clear, coherent or convincing vision of the early Dodd and the adult Dodd as a consequence remains ambiguous. He insists that he has a great deal of love to give, not merely on stage in contact with hundreds and thousands but personally. Yet the fact remains that he has remained a relatively isolated figure which is surprising for someone who insists that his childhood was a very happy one, that he was well provided for materially and emotionally, that life is full of wonderful, joyful experiences. But, argue some listeners, what is Clare going on about? Everyone doesn't have to have a close personal relationship, does not have to have children, can live a perfectly fulfilled life in relative solitude particularly if, like Ken Dodd, they have satisyfing, rewarding, respected careers. Just because he is married and has children does not mean that anyone who isn't needs explaining!

These are legitimate objections but they miss the point. Ken Dodd on a number of occasions came close to marriage. On at least one the woman involved wanted to marry him. But he never did and the reason he gives me, that he was too busy, seems to me somewhat unconvincing to say the least. Perhaps Ken Dodd's desire to retain control of his life and circumstances proved too strong – when eventually I can provoke him to desist from idealising women and identify some faults he picks on the way that women can nag, pick on the weak spots, make demands. Because by and large he tends to praise motherhood, women, his parents, family life in near-extravagant terms, the few occasions when the guard appears to slip merit attention – his irritable aside on the demands of 'the family', his admission that many people in show-business are dreadful businessmen, his concluding regretful wish that he had expressed his feelings more.

There is a considerable emphasis in the Dodd interview on the need for self-reliance, independence, doing it on your own. Even in his reflections on God and a spiritual dimension to his life, there is a marked emphasis on his doing something special, some lonely, redemptive mission. Ken Dodd started life as a salesman, as someone who has to survive, earn a living on his ability to persuade, manipulate, find a weakness, a need, a vulnerability. A comedian on stage is in a not dissimilar relationship with his audience. Ken Dodd's vision of the world, of the adult world, like that of many comics, is a lonely at times even hostile one. His humour harks back to a child's world full of magic, unpredictability, glorious anarchy and mystery. Such people are not easy to live with – nor interview as I discovered for myself.

CLARE: Ken Dodd, O.B.E. was born on November 8th 1930, in Knotty Ash, Liverpool. His father was a coal merchant and Ken Dodd worked in the family business and then as a salesman of pots, polishes, potions and lotions before taking his first steps as a stand-up comedian. In September 1954 he made his professional debut at The Empire Theatre in Nottingham. The following year saw the first of many a summer season at Blackpool and he was a national star by 1965, when, after a record-breaking forty-two weeks at the London Palladium, he was elected Showbusiness Personality of the Year by the Variety Club of Great Britain. Since then he has made a number of hit records, starred as Malvolio in *Twelfth Night*, has made several Royal Command Performances and is now a veteran of radio and television. In his book entitled *How tickled I am* the critic Michael Billington declares 'Dodd is too manic, too fervent, too irresistibly and overwhelmingly funny to be other than England's undisputed clown prince'.

CLARE: Ken Dodd, you clearly enjoy tremendously entertaining thousands, indeed millions, how do you feel about talking about yourself?

DODD: Well delighted, delighted, because to coin a phrase I'd say I was full of plumptiousness and feeling, well completely discumknockerated actually because when you invited me to talk about myself I tried to think well, 'What will I say, how will I approach it, how will I answer him?' A lot of people are frank, very very frank, very blunt, brutally frank and they try to be really honest. Other times your mind is ticking over and you say you know this would sound good, if I say this, this will sound good. So I don't know which way to answer you, I shall try and be a mixture I think. I think I'll try and be honest.

CLARE: In general I've noted in the various things you've said and things that have been written about you that by and large you're a private person.

DODD: Yes I think so. I'm definitely several layers and yes, a private person. At the same time you know I like to show off now and again, of course I do. I've got some opinions which I'm quite prepared to stand on my little soap-box and let fly.

CLARE: If you were to say to me well why have I asked to interview you I think one reason is your occupation, and I'll come back to that in a minute, the other is that I also note in the things that are written about you that you yourself are quite interested in the psychology of humour.

DODD: Very, deeply interested.

CLARE: You have read a good deal about it. And what I thought I'd do, because you and I know time is scarce, is to look at you, if you like, to try and make sense of various attempts that people have made to explain the kind of thing you do.

DODD: Yes, I started in 1954 and I was a salesman at the time, selling things. I've always sold things. I've always dealt with the public, first of all knocking on doors and dealing with customers. I think that's where 'the missus' came from — 'By Jove missus' — and then when I turned professional comedian I wanted to know what it was I was selling. So I started just going to libraries and looking up the words 'laughter', 'comedy', 'comedian', 'comic', 'clown'. I was the sort of boy who used to read avidly. I could read when I was four and I used to read books and books, and particularly adventure books. I wanted life to be an adventure. I wanted to be an explorer, a pioneer. So here was a land that was uncharted. Here was a land that had never been explained before. Aristotle, I think, said that the essence of the comic was a buckled mill-wheel and I can understand that now. I couldn't understand it then, but I can understand it now, meaning it's life a little bit wobbly.

CLARE: In putting together your own model of yourself you point already to two things. You point to the fact that you were in the business of selling, your father was a merchant and you were a seller. You point to the fact that as a child you had great interest in the fantastical and the wondrous and the wonderful. Was there anything else in the early Dodd childhood? You were one of how many?

DODD: I've got an older brother and a younger sister.

CLARE: So you were in the middle.

DODD: Yes, and we had a very very happy childhood. The funniest man I ever knew was Arthur Dodd, my father. He was a brilliant clown. He knew some great stories. I still tell stories now, jokes that my father, well his father told him.

CLARE: Really. If I'd seen you as an eight-year-old, a ten-year-old, a twelve-year-old, was there that about you?

DODD: Oh no, no.

CLARE: What were you like?

DODD: Quite shy actually, quite shy and quite meek and mild.

CLARE: There is about a lot of comedy a regression. It is a

negative word, a return to childhood. In fact it's the endorse-
ment of childhood values, of fun, of anarchy, of colour in a
grey and dull world.

DODD: I think everyone is born with a spirit of play in them
and I think as the various pressures come on you as you
grow older then some people, very unfortunately, inhibit
that spirit of play and a lot of that playfulness goes out of
their life which is a shame really.

CLARE: Did it happen to you? Were attempts made?

DODD: Oh I think so yes, lots of attempts have been made.

CLARE: By whom?

DODD: All sorts of people – schoolteachers, rates officers. But
to most people who are comedy-minded, discipline comes
very hard, is very difficult.

CLARE: You say that with a certain feeling.

DODD: Yes, well . . .

CLARE: In your case what sort of discipline?

DODD: I don't take kindly to it I'm sorry to say. I know a lot of
it's for my own good. Well they say it is, over the years,
schoolteachers have told me you know. My headmaster,
Bonky Bill, who was the first one at the junior school and
then later I passed a scholarship to a grammar school and
went to the Holt in Liverpool. Yes, I'm afraid so, I was always
in trouble.

CLARE: Were you? How would this show up in your, in your
personal characteristics? Does it mean that you're less constrained by things like time?

DODD: Ah that was very tactful, that was very tactful of you.

CLARE: Why?

DODD: Oh, I'm sorry, I thought you'd heard about me, I'm not
the most punctual person in the world.

CLARE: Another theory, of course, of humour is Freud's theory
of splitting it into innocent and tendentious. Innocent
humour, if we just take that for a second, you very beauti-
fully illustrate. That's to say those jokes that are based round
worlds like 'plumptiousness' and 'tattifilarious.'

DODD: That is whimsy.

CLARE: Whimsy — the word associations, the punning and so on.

DODD: I think a lot of the problem when philosophers and psychologists and psychiatrists try to explain humour is that they will treat it as one formula whereas you wouldn't expect to explain music, the word 'music' with one pat formula.

CLARE: What about when you are low? I suppose the most persistent idea, certainly widespread amongst the public, is the idea of a melancholic comic?

DODD: The Pagliacci. No I don't think so.

CLARE: You aren't too happy with the notion of Pagliacci, but at the same time neither are you suggesting to me, are you, that you're not a man without flesh and blood like everyone else?

DODD: No. I remember when my mother passed away I was dreading it, but it was totally different to what one would expect.

CLARE: In what way?

DODD: Well, I once again knew that I was helped because I didn't fall into this tremendous trough of despair, I didn't go all to pieces. I felt some strength come from somewhere.

CLARE: From where? Where do you draw your strength from?

DODD: I don't know, I don't know, I don't know where this strength came from. I have an idea but . . .

CLARE: Well what would you say?

DODD: No, well it, it's, it's wrong for me to . . .

CLARE: You're not referring to someone else? You're referring to some kind of religious source of support?

DODD: I think so, yes, I think so.

CLARE: How religious are you? Are you a very religious man?

DODD: Yes, yes, I think so, yes. I think I try to have conversations with my maker. I find it difficult sometimes to find some religious services relevant to our world of 1987. I find them a little bit medieval and therefore sometimes I have to make my own dialogues up and I make my own conversations, but in that respect yes I do, and I pray . . .

CLARE: When your mother died was that the source of support? Or was it something stronger than that?

DODD: It was very, very strong. It was very, very strong, and I was able to go on and do my next show and I remember it was a very, very good show. I was, you know, I was really moved to tears and in taking this applause at the same time I was crying with, I don't know, relief, joy, that I knew they were there with me.

CLARE: So you're saying in a sense that on stage, doing what you do, you were able to in some way what? Not exorcise, but express your grief?

DODD: No I think I was helped. Yes I think I was helped directly.

CLARE: Directly helped?

DODD: Directly helped, yes, I'm not a spiritualist.

CLARE: No. This is divine. This would be an assistance from God himself?

DODD: I don't know, I don't know.

CLARE: How else has it happened to you? Have you had other similar experiences?

DODD: Many times yes, yes many times. But I believe, I believe in it. I believe that I am helped quite a lot.

CLARE: In other ways, in other areas?

DODD: Oh yes. Well certainly in my profession.

CLARE: I'm interested how people, at crisis points in their lives, what it is they derive support from. Because after all, as I've often explained to others, I see a lot of people who are casualties. Now you've survived in a sense.

DODD: Oh, yes, but I think you have to be also self-supportive as well. If I have a guardian angel, if God is looking after me, I don't want to be bothering them all the time, you know. Every time I get a parking ticket, every time I want to get through a traffic jam, I don't all of a sudden, I don't start screaming for help. But there are occasions when you do need, you feel perhaps a little extra, a little extra confidence would come in handy.

CLARE: And it is a strikingly solitary life, the comic, on stage. The stand-up, the man on his own.

DODD: Being a comedian, being a live comedian is a wonderful, wonderful experience. I don't know what it is but there certainly is some kind of magic that happens, some magic thing happens that transforms you from being a very ordinary person like me. I go on the stage there and I feel like twenty feet tall because here this audience are all laughing away and everybody happy, and they're all laughing and their eyes are shining and they want to applaud and I really feel wonderful. It's a wonderful experience.

CLARE: Is it the best?

DODD: The best experience? Oh I don't know about that. Life is full of such wonderful, joyful experiences. I mean you can get a high, I think, in your life just walking through a garden and seeing all the beautiful flowers, and particularly if it's just been raining, it can actually make you almost keel over in ecstasy. There are also wonderful experiences, other experiences in life which can make you shout out in ecstasy.

CLARE: You said something, somewhere, once, about the things that you were touching on that made people laugh. One of the things you talked about was 'man's delight in women, women's contempt for men.' I was rather intrigued by that. It sort of reminded me of Don McGill postcards and so on.

DODD: Well, I think yes, I think man's delight with ladies is absolutely the most wonderful thing, isn't it? I mean ladies are so beautiful and so marvellous and wonderful, oh!

CLARE: Why did you never marry one?

DODD: To be honest with you, I was, as you know, I was engaged for a long time. But I came into showbusiness in 54 and to be honest I know it sounds amazing but we were too busy, we were so busy. Every show that came along and every challenge, every television series that came along posed this fresh set of emotional challenges.

CLARE: When you say 'we,' you're talking about yourself and your fiancée.

DODD: Yes, yes.

CLARE: Anita.

DODD: Yes.

CLARE: Did she want to get married?

DODD: Oh, yes, oh, yes, it was quite normal you know, but I mean everything was normal but . . .

CLARE: You never did.

DODD: We were always too busy.

CLARE: And it lasted, how long?

DODD: Oh quite a while, quite a long time.

CLARE: Well, ten years, twelve, I mean I have no idea?

DODD: It lasted a long time, a long time, but there you go. But now when you say 'women's contempt for men' I think what I meant by that was that, well, they don't always get a very easy life do they and so I think their way of . . .

CLARE: Well do they?

DODD: Many a lady saying caustic remarks about her husband and all sorts of remarks, but they love them really, you know they really are loyal to them, but they can't help, you know, firing off an occasional salvo now and again, yes.

CLARE: Was that something you worried about?

DODD: Oh, I noticed.

CLARE: Did you worry that that's what would become of a relationship you might have?

DODD: Oh, no, no I think men deserve to be hammered now and again, of course I do. We're terrible to ladies. It's a man's world, isn't it?

CLARE: I don't know, I'm asking you.

DODD: Oh yes, it's a man's world, yes. We get the best, we get the best of everything, oh, we get the best of everything.

CLARE: Was it that when you say you were too busy?

DODD: Look, what you get, when you get a really good relationship with a woman you get everything don't you? You get a wife, a lover, a mother, you get the lot all in one. And what do they get?

CLARE: What do they get?

DODD: Poof! A man generally gets crabbier as he grows older doesn't he, gets more, more demanding, more selfish? Some men, you can't generalise, you can't generalise, but . . .

CLARE: That's certainly there in your humour.

DODD: Oh yes, yes. You see, you have these, I think your

word, your word, academically, is 'ambivalent' isn't it? We all have these dual feelings about each other.

CLARE: Would you be ambivalent about women?

DODD: Ladies can, they can get on your nerves at times, you know they, they have this natural ability to give you hell if they want to. If they really want something doing like, you know, if they want something, a shelf putting up or a garden digging they can, by jove they know how to, they know all the weak spots.

CLARE: What was your mother like, because you mention her?

DODD: Oh, absolutely lovely, absolutely wonderful, a great sense of humour, she was marvellous. She used to say, 'You can do anything you want to do if you want to hard enough, you can be anyone, be prime minister.'

CLARE: I'm puzzled Ken, about the fact that you didn't get married, because it's clear from what you've said and I think from the little I've read about you that, that you like women and you met this woman, you knew her for years, you had a good mother . . .

DODD: I have a lady now who I love very much.

CLARE: You do?

DODD: Yes, no, I think I want to be a toy boy, no (laugh). The first time when I was engaged I was trying to become a name, I was trying to get to the top of the bill. I always wanted to be a star. I love being a star. I love being a comedian. I love being Ken Dodd. I would like to be an international star, oh, yes.

CLARE: What is it about being a star?

DODD: It's an overworked word of course. What it means to be a success is the word, to be a success. How do you mean what is it?

CLARE: Just that, what is its appeal?

DODD: Oh it's a wonderful feeling, it means you've succeeded. It means you've succeeded, you've developed skill, you've tried, you've worked at it.

CLARE: How single-minded do you have to be?

DODD: Very, very. You have to put a lot of things to one side, oh yes. I think in my lifetime I think I've only been to about three football matches, three or four, oh yes, oh yes, oh yes.

CLARE: Do you ever not work? Do you ever take a holiday?

DODD: Oh yes, very much so, yes.

CLARE: Completely? What do you do when you do?

DODD: Well we went just recently to Majorca, got five bad days and two good ones and spent most of the time eating.

CLARE: So you can take time out?

DODD: Oh yes. Then again there's two different kinds of holidays. There's one where you lie down and try to recharge your batteries and the other one where you need a holiday for the mind. Then I try to go to one of the capital cities for one of these breaks there, you know, and go to somewhere like Vienna or Berlin, Paris, these are the places I've been to, you know, so working my way round those.

CLARE: Do you have withdrawal symptoms from work, do you mind it?

DODD: I'd be telling you a fib if I said that I didn't. When I go on holiday I can't help liking sometimes little kids on the beach coming and saying, coming and staring at me and wanting me to sign their postcards. And I do like ladies and gentlemen on holiday, particularly if they're getting on in years, looking at me and saying − 'It's Ken Dodd.' I do like that yes, I do like it, yes.

CLARE: You like children?

DODD: Oh yes, I love children yes, yes I grew up with them. I went to school with them (laugh), yes, of course I do. Children have this wonderful sort of, well it is wonderful, because it's wondrous the way they look at the world. It's so unspoiled, it's so fresh and new, and you can tell it's all new to them so I wouldn't do anything ever to sort of taint it or disappoint it. I like to be nice to all children. I like to sign their books for them and I like to make them feel as though that was a good moment because I like to be, I like to be Ken Dodd the comedian, the entertainer, the showbusiness fella, yes.

CLARE: But you're not a fountain of fun and happiness, you're presumably a difficult man as well?

DODD: Yes I can be, that's right, yes, I must admit I like my own way, yes, yes.

CLARE: That's what people say?

DODD: Yes, do they?

CLARE: I'm asking you.

DODD: Oh, no I don't think so, no, I don't think it's got about, I don't think the word's got about (laugh).

CLARE: But why did you say it?

DODD: Well because you see in showbusiness, particularly in television and, and on the stage as well, when there's a producer then the trouble with producers is they will produce, they can't leave it alone. The trouble with producers of a light entertainment show, whether it's on the stage or television, they have to get their not four pen'orth but nine pen'orth in. It's all they want. They want all the feathers and the spangles and they won't let the people who've been booked to juggle and be funny get on with it. They obscure it with lights and mirrors and smoke bombs and so on.

CLARE: I mean in general you like to control your world?

DODD: Yes, yes, yes.

CLARE: In all its areas, really?

DODD: Very much so, yes, very much so. I don't take too kindly to being told 'Stand on that chalk mark.' I think most art is very, very spoiled you know, really, you know you get all this applause and people keep forcing money into your hand.

CLARE: Yes, you are I suppose very spoiled – everything revolves round you.

DODD: When I think of the way my father used to have to work, when I think of the way I used to have to work, and then all of a sudden I found this wonderful thing, if I went on and said 'By Jove, how tickled I am,' and everybody said 'good old Ken, here poof, have this,' which is marvellous, wonderful. But I'm very interested in the way my mind works and the way other people's minds work. I'm a dabbler in psychology. I'm a great one for trying to find why people do things.

CLARE: People are interested because they want to change the way they're doing things for the future. Other people are interested because they're interested in making sense of the past. In your case, which is it? You tend to look to psychology as a way of increasing your control?

DODD: Oh, yes, because I think the secret of happiness is to invest I think in the future and see something happen, oh yes. The past? The past can be fascinating. You can look at Stonehenge and think, by jove, think of those druids pulling those things across Salisbury Plain, praying for somebody to invent lego!

CLARE: Ah, yes, I was thinking of *your* past.

DODD: Oh, I see, sorry.

CLARE: Not so much the druids.

DODD: Oh, my past, oh, well my past, well I don't know.

CLARE: When you look back, what puzzles you most looking back about yourself?

DODD: About me? I don't think anything does. I'm very ordinary aren't I, look at me, very ordinary, very ordinary.

CLARE: Well not that ordinary. I mean there's the hair!

DODD: Oh, sitting here in my Marks and Spencer's suit. Oh, the hair bit.

CLARE: The stick, the language, the manic flow.

DODD: The hair bit started quite accidentally. When I first turned professional I was too busy to have my hair cut, to be honest with you.

CLARE: You know that's the second time you've used 'too busy' as an explanation for why you don't do something!

DODD: Yes, I was too busy to have my hair cut.

CLARE: If you're too busy to do something, it really means that it's relatively low on your list of priorities.

DODD: Oh, no I don't think . . .

CLARE: Yes it is you know. Now when you said to me 'too busy to get your hair cut,' 'too busy to get married,' doesn't it mean that in your list of priorities it wasn't high enough because you would do it if you wanted to do it. You said your mother told you that.

DODD: Oh, I know I can tell you.

CLARE: 'If you want to do it you'll do it.'

DODD: Oh, there's another expression, 'It wasn't necessary.'

CLARE: Wasn't necessary?

DODD: No, it wasn't necessary. It wasn't necessary for me to have my hair cut and it wasn't really necessary for me to . . .

CLARE: Though you came from a family and clearly family is an important institution to you, you're quite a conservative with a small and maybe even a big 'C' but it's an important institution — now don't go off on that for a minute, come back, I can see you going off . . .

DODD: Family is a great thing although, although it does annoy me sometimes when the emphasis is placed on 'the families', — you know you'd think that people who either live on their own or separately don't exist. Everything must happen for 'the family.' There are other people in the world as well you know but, you're quite right, yes I do, I do love to see families and I do think the family is a wonderful thing and I'm very close to my brother and sister and I was very close to my mother and father, yes.

CLARE: Did you ever feel the need to have that yourself? I'm very struck reading you about this, because you've said it on a number of occasions about your father's marvellous ability to make you laugh and the family tea, did you ever want that for children of your own?

DODD: I'm very fond of dogs, I love dogs, I can't be without a dog, I love dogs. Our little dog's just been barred from coming in now, they won't let him in the BBC. I have a great deal of love to give out to little people. Yes you could have a point, yes I think I, yes I would, yes I'd dearly love, yes of course I would, but I was too busy. You've got a thing about this haven't you?

CLARE: I'm interested. Why did you think I have a thing about it? You said something about if you want to do something you'll do it, that is a philosophy.

DODD: No my mother said it.

CLARE: Your mother said it, but you clearly admired her.

DODD: My mother said if you want to be a success at something, if you really try hard enough you will and I wanted, I desperately wanted to be a success on the stage in showbusiness, I really did, I still do. I eat, sleep and dream it, yes I do.

CLARE: Are you difficult to live with?

DODD: I don't think so, no, no I have, like most people, I have my funny little ways. No I don't think so, I'm very untidy, very untidy yes. I'm a hoarder of anything, newspapers, magazines, 'don't throw that out.'

CLARE: Are you a hoarder of money?

DODD: Oh no, no, well I like money, why have you got some? (laugh)

CLARE: You made a crack, I think it was on the Save the Children's Telethon when they got a hundred quid out of you, you said something like 'you know how difficult that is,' or something, I wondered?

DODD: Oh yes, oh yes, well I'm a businessman, I'm a business-man. A businessman means — yes you're quite right to pick that up because a lot of entertainers, particularly light entertainment people, are absolutely abysmal when it comes to handling money. They're absolutely dreadful and that's why they're always in trouble. You know they're always, you know, bankrupt or they let other people look after their money and I won't do this. You see, once again, I try to do everything myself with my father being a coal merchant and having respect for money at an early age, knowing what it could do and what lack of it can do.

CLARE: So you were always someone who was going to control that side of things.

DODD: Oh, I knew the value of money. Even at an early age I could see how hard my parents were working and we always had the best of food and the lovely Christmas presents and birthday presents. It really was a lovely, a lovely childhood, I couldn't fault it at all, absolutely wonderful.

CLARE: Have you an unhappy memory?

DODD: Of childhood? No, I only ever had one unhappy feeling that every now and again used to overwhelm me and that was the idea that one day I would have to lose my mother and father and that's the one thing that used to frighten me, yes.

CLARE: What was it like when you did lose them?

DODD: Terrible, terrible, absolutely. I thought it was going to be terrible you know, I thought, you know the looking, the dreading it and seeing it gradually unrelentingly moving towards me. I think you know you pray, you try and make bargains, you try and do deals with God, but you know it's not going to happen, and then when it did I thought, well you know that's it then, it would be like the whole thing will open up, the ground will open up and I'll just go down into it and that'll be the end of it, you know.

CLARE: What about when your fiancée died?

DODD: Same, same thing yes, yes same thing, yes.

CLARE: That had been a long illness and were you around that time having to go on stage?

DODD: Yes, yes, yes.

CLARE: Did you ever lose faith?

DODD: In God? Yes, yes.

CLARE: Is that the kind of thing that would provoke it or was it over something else?

DODD: Oh, no it was over that. You know if you, if you ask someone, if you knock at a door and nobody answers you tend to think there's nobody home.

CLARE: Do you think that you've got a special vocation, mission, that there's a purpose?

DODD: Yes I do actually, yes, yes I do. I think part of it has been fulfilled. I think part of my reason for being alive, I think there is a reason for everyone, and I think there's a reason for most things. I think part of my reason for being alive, I get an absolutely wonderful reaction from people. You get some marvellous feedback from the people who you've entertained and you think, good God and I mean good God, did I really, was I really able to help that person, that's wonderful, that's fantastic, that is wonderful. Oh, that is, that makes me really feel good, that makes me feel as though I'm doing something. Perhaps I've got a reason then, I've got a purpose in life, I'm not just a dot, not just a speck. And then maybe, perhaps it's just the thing that keeps you going. I do feel that there is yet something, yes there's something I've got to do.

CLARE: Do you know what it is?

DODD: No I don't, no I don't know what it is. I don't know what it is.

CLARE: Do you want to know?

DODD: Yes because I want to do it properly.

CLARE: What do you think it might be?

DODD: I don't know, I don't know.

CLARE: But it's a feeling you have?

DODD: Yes, yes, maybe the feeling when you're a child sometimes you feel that you're special.

CLARE: Did you?

DODD: Yes.

CLARE: From the word go. Were you treated special?

DODD: I think yes, of course, as I say I had absolutely wonderful parents.

CLARE: But of the three children were you special? Would they say you were?

DODD: I don't think so, no. I'm sure they wouldn't, no.

CLARE: But you felt you were special. Why?

DODD: It may go back to the fact that when I was about a year old, I think I was about a year, eighteen months old, I nearly popped off because I had a very nasty dose of double pneumonia and I nearly didn't make it.

CLARE: Were your parents religious?

DODD: My mother was, yes my mother was. I don't know about my father. I think, yes I think so, although I think he'd had a hard life, my dad, he was getting a bit cynical I think, about it all.

CLARE: I wondered whether in your survival did either of them convey to you a notion that there was something special about this, that you'd survived through the double pneumonia?

DODD: Well I know they had someone in to say prayers over me, I know that, they always said, they always regarded that as a miracle, yes.

CLARE: Right. So you have had that sense about yourself.

DODD: When I was a little boy I used to really believe that I really was, I was going to do something worthwhile.

CLARE: But you still do think that.

DODD: Oh yes, only in a different way now.

CLARE: So that there's something else?

DODD: Yes I think it's something.

CLARE: Politics?

DODD: No, no, no I think it's something deeper than that, I think it's something, I don't know what it is. It may be something that won't mean anything to anybody else, but maybe I will affect someone's life somewhere, maybe I've got to do something.

CLARE: Yes. It's been a good life in many ways.

DODD: Hey, wait a minute, whoa!

CLARE: Have you any regrets?

DODD: I've regretted there's no more of it, yes. I want to be shot by a jealous husband at the age of a hundred and twenty.

CLARE: That's I suppose as good a way of going out as any but, looking back, have you any regrets?

DODD: Oh yes, lots of regrets.

CLARE: Any major one?

DODD: Oh yes I wish I'd been a better son to my mother and father. I wish I'd have told them many many more times. We weren't a sort of a sloppy family, a demonstrative family, but I wish I'd have told them how much they meant to me. I wish, yes, I wish I'd have had children. I wish I had a lot more confidence. I wish I wasn't so terrified sometimes when, you know, if you do a big, big show, like in the Royal Variety Performances, that is it that really separates the men from the boys, and I'm one of the boys.

Sir Peter Hall

Setting up the interview with Sir Peter Hall took some doing. He never seemed to be where he was supposed to be, he appeared to be doing three mammoth undertakings at one and the same time and yet it was clear that he was not only agreeable to the interview but was genuinely helpful in various efforts to make it happen. Since the interview nothing very much has changed. As I write this I learn that Sir Peter, now married for a fourth time, is in Manhattan writing not one but two film scripts, is rising at 6.a.m. every day to tap his memoirs into a word processor and is directing a Broadway play. His new wife, keen clearly to match this prolific productivity, is expecting a child, Hall's sixth.

He tells me he is appalled at the pressure he puts himself under, the punishing pace at which he works and lives. It is extraordinary. He produces and directs plays, operas, television serials, he keeps and publishes a detailed diary, he has run the National Theatre, has had three wives, and hates to waste a single minute, hates to be too early for anything, hates to stand still, worries that someday nobody might want him.

So the central question that slowly emerges in this interview is what lies behind this compulsive, greedy need to have it all, to achieve, to do? A chemical addiction — certainly that plays its part. Sir Peter enjoys the highs he experiences from all that adrenalin running around in his veins — but that only goes to raise another question. What caused the addiction?

Sir Peter Hall started with a very good family matrix for the ultimate design of a high-achieving male adult. His parents believed in the puritan work ethic, in the importance, the crucial importance of education in empowering a child to take control of his adult life, in getting on and achieving security, emotional, professional, financial. He was an only child with a soft, gentle, intelligent father and a highly ambitious mother. It was Freud who once observed 'a man who has been the indisputable favourite of his mother keeps for life the feeling of a conqueror, that confidence of success that often induces real success' and he, being the undisputed favourite of his doting mother, was well placed to know. Peter Hall, however, was not just the favourite of his mother but of a veritable legion of grandfathers and grandmothers, uncles and aunts who would appear to have regarded this promising, talented, energetic young man with considerable hope and affection.

Sir Peter Hall exudes that confident belief that he is a leader, he is of interest, he has something to say that warrants being heard that children with talent and an ambitious background take absolutely for granted. Yet there is of course a parallel anxiety. There is the burden of other men's hopes. There is the loneliness of the achievement. As any success that occurs is yours and yours alone, so is the failure. Sir Peter Hall identifies as yet another of the spurs to further action the anxiety of failure and oblivion – Graham Greene once observed with characteristic mordant gloom that success is only delayed failure. This greed for achievement, like any other greed, cannot be satisfied. To that extent Hall is insatiable. He can only keep going.

'Why do you work so hard Papa? What are you trying to prove?' The questions are those of his son, Christopher, then aged ten. They are, as his father admits, extraordinarily apt. Sir Peter Hall denies he is trying to prove anything and the extent that his denials are convincing have to be left to his children, wives, listeners and readers to judge. But there are surely grounds for doubt. He is not driven by a need to dominate others – although dissenting voices can be heard. Others had told me of a mercurial, grandiose side to Hall's nature. There is John Osborne's much-quoted description of Hall as Dr Fu Manchu, the dictator of the National Theatre. There were the fiery public disagreements with his succession of equally powerful wives – actress Leslie Caron, opera diva Maria Ewing and former secretary, Jacqueline Taylor. It is interesting to note that when in an interview in the *Sunday Times* with Geordie Grieg (1 March 1992) he speaks of his relationship with his fourth wife, Nikki, it is her 'non-jealous and non-interventionist sense' that merits his praise.

I do not know whether Sir Peter Hall recognises the extent to which there can be no room in his immediate world for an ego and a drive as demanding, massive and assertive as his own. It is surely worth noting that he chose early on to be a director – a role which ensures that his working situation will never be short of gargantuan egos and voracious narcissists but by virtue of his role he will be in control of them and not the other way around. He is clearly attracted to and by people with a comparable energy and ambition – such personalities often are. Such attraction can lead to marriage with rarely successful results. Of his three marriages, the one that lasted longest involved a woman who was not herself a star or performer but had played a key supporting role to Hall's own professional career. But even that did not last. There is a moment in the interview when Sir Peter Hall, in something of an aside, protests, 'I'm sure that I try to make sacrifices but I can't not be what I want to be' – the contradiction in the statement is left hanging and not confronted. But he does recognise that he is very demanding, impatient of others not as committed to doing as he is, stimulated by the challenge inherent in motivating others to do one's own will.

What makes Sir Peter Hall a stimulating interview subject is that he brought his passion, energy and drive right into the studio and for the couple of hours that we were together his concentration was total. God knows what else he had on that day and week. I have come to recognise that single-minded ability as one of the marks of achievers – the ability to block out everything that is extraneous to the task in hand. Whether it is in-born, or environmentally cultivated I do not know. But in Hall's case both may have operated. It is an evocative picture he paints of his childhood at the tiny railway station in Barnham and the small, precocious boy being excused the washing-up to read 'a serious book'. Reading serious books has excused Hall the washing-up many times since.

What if Sir Peter Hall were to stop? Why would he? The one

unpredictable element in the life of people such as Hall is health – his talent, which he worries about, is too manifold and multi-faceted to let him down at this stage but body and mind are less resilient. He is wise enough to recognise that self-sufficient as he is and has been all his life he cannot manage on his own. He needs someone with whom to share not primarily the success but the doubts. Without such support it is not too fanciful to suggest that he could become depressed. He talks of it. He has experienced it. He is temperamentally prone to it. His massive investment of energy in living combats the tendency and effectively keeps it at bay. He does not want to stop, does not want to waste precious time. He has a painfully acute awareness of mortality, time running out, death – there is never a day, he says, when he does not think about it, the pain, the fury and the suffering. For some, such an acute sense of mortality is enough to render them immobile, paralysed by indecision and ruminations on the seeming purposelessness. For Hall it is one more spur to action.

The microphone switched off, Sir Peter Hall looks at me expectantly and asks, as so many interviewees do of their interviewers, 'Is that what you wanted?' Then off he rushes to keep death at bay and everyone else under control.

CLARE: Sir Peter Hall was born on November 22nd 1930, the son of a railway goods clerk and a draper's assistant. An only and a gifted child, he won a scholarship to grammar school and then went on to St Catherine's College, Cambridge, where he read English. From an early age he wanted to be a theatre director and his life has seen that ambition amply fulfilled. He founded the Royal Shakespeare Company, was director of the National Theatre, succeeding Laurence Olivier in 1973, was artistic director of the Glyndebourne Festival Opera, and he's now running his own company. For services to the theatre he was awarded the CBE and in 1977 was knighted. He's been married and divorced three times and has five children.

CLARE: Sir Peter, why do you do this interview? Are you particularly interested in yourself?

HALL: I was actually very resistant to doing this interview, I lead a busy life and it was difficult to fit in and I was glad. It was difficult to say no, but finally I was asked so many times that I thought I'd better do it. Because it represents something that I don't like but which I have to do which is making oneself a public figure and the reason you do that finally is because if you exist and work in a public media it sells tickets. I am called by my friends and at my best I am a 'name director'. I don't mean that I sell as many tickets as great actors but I sell some. The public over thirty-five years have seen a lot of my work so they come because I sign it. This is part of making sure they know about me.

CLARE: Are there any other motives? Take for example the fact that you published your own diaries?

HALL: Yes well that was actually for the same reason as I'm here now. I kept the diaries not for publication. PR and publicity person John Goodwin at the National Theatre thought it would be quite useful for people to understand what doing that job entailed and persuaded me to publish them. It was successful. The publisher then asked me to do a regular kind of two- or three-year diaries and I found I couldn't. Once I knew it was for public consumption it inhibited me so I haven't kept a diary since.

CLARE: Nonetheless you're not a man to do anything that you don't want to do. In that sense although the explanation you've given me to some extent suggests a certain reluctance, bowing to others' persuasion, the little I know of you and read about you suggests a man who would not bow unless at the end of the day, he decided he wanted to do it?

HALL: I hope that I do what I believe in. I hope I stand up for what I believe in and I certainly know that in my profession it's no good doing anything you don't believe in because I can't do it. I mean you have to have a subjective and instinctive engagement with the play or opera or film that you're directing because otherwise you cannot actually create and that's very difficult to define. But this whole publicising oneself question, talking all about oneself, I really do find extremely difficult. It is the classic cliché isn't it that all movie stars say they don't like talking about themselves and then proceed to talk about themselves. We always say we don't like talking about ourselves, but I actually am very shy, I don't like public life very much, I don't like parties, I don't like public gatherings. I think that's partly the reason I'm a director.

CLARE: In those situations you describe, parties, would the shyness cause you physical distress, anxiety?

HALL: Yes, a feeling of awkwardness and perspiration, tension, yes, yes. It's paradoxical I know, because in a sense I spend my whole working life in social conditions, with groups of very highly motivated egotistical people. Again it may be why I do it. I've noticed that many performers are very shy, many actors are terribly shy people. The popular idea of the actor as a show-off is not actually usually true. I also don't think directors are show-offs.

CLARE: So when you for example read your own diaries for publication and saw your life laid out, as seen by you, laid out in front of you, did that make you feel more curious about yourself?

HALL: No it actually fairly appalled me, the pressure I put myself under. Also, I didn't quite recognise myself but then I don't think you do recognise yourself, either when you hear yourself speaking or you see yourself talking on television or when you read a diary. I think I should just explain about the diary because it sounds a bit off for somebody who's published his innermost thoughts about running a theatre to say I don't like being public. I actually thought that I was living through such an extraordinary time opening the National Theatre that I would simply dictate every morning at six o'clock what had happened the day before into a dictaphone and then had it typed out. I would never read it and I would never look back at it, so it is as honest as I could make it the day after, and it's inconsistent and it's full of contradictions as a consequence. The selection of it was done by John Goodwin.

CLARE: But you said when you read it you were appalled at the pressures you put yourself under. Just say a little about that.

HALL: It was getting up at six in the morning and finishing at eleven or twelve at night, spending a great deal of time on administration, having four or five hours of peace, in a sense, in the rehearsal room, where you weren't disturbed and then coming out to a round of meetings and almost certainly seeing a performance in the evening. It was a tough life, physically and emotionally. It was a bit like being at war.

CLARE: Were you any clearer, having read it, as to why you did it?

HALL: It's possibly chemical. My doctor tells me I'm an adrenalin addict. My system needs a lot of adrenalin and produces a lot of adrenalin. Therefore I love stress and it's that balancing act of, I suppose, seeking stress and yet not wanting to have too much stress that one's got to try. There's also the fact that I like achieving. I'm sure that goes back to my parents who believed passionately in trying to get on in the world. I had an extremely ambitious mother and an extremely unambitious father, but a very wise father, who had no ambition whatsoever.

CLARE: What was he like? Your father.

HALL: Very very gentle, very very warm, very intelligent. He was the first one of the family who had gone to secondary school. He was a scholarship boy, and he went on the railways and in the thirties, this was the late twenties when he started, the railways were a very assured occupation. At a time of increasing unemployment, if you were a railwayman you were all right. I remember my father earning three pounds ten a week and it was very hard. We had very very little money but he had security and as I say he had very little ambition. He was musical, he could sing quite well, he'd been in the Bury St Edmunds Amateur Operatic Society and he was wise and tolerant, he loved nature. My happiest memories as a child, when I was around six or seven, we lived at a tiny railway station on the borders of Suffolk and Norfolk called Barnham, long since gone, which had four trains a day, four passenger trains a day, and a goods train at lunchtime and a signalman and an odd job man and my father and we lived over the platform. There was no electricity, no gas, an outside loo, no bathroom but we were in the heart of the country and my father looked after the platform gardens all day and then put his hat on when the train came in. I think that was probably his happiest time too. My mother by contrast was extremely ambitious for herself and extremely frustrated that my father wasn't more ambitious, and extremely ambitious for me. They did spoil me in that from my earliest years if I wanted to read a book, providing it was what they called a serious book, I was excused the washing-up. I was always allowed to have the space and the time to read, to study. They started me on piano lessons when I was six years old which I think was sixpence a week, which was, you know, a considerable sum for them, and everything stopped if I wanted to practise the piano.

CLARE: You were an only child?

HALL: I was an only child, I wished passionately that I wasn't. Yes I did and do. My mother always said to me 'We couldn't do for two what we can do for one.' Whether that was true or not I don't know.

CLARE: But you wished then and you do still, because?

HALL: Because it was lonely. I still am lonely. I still feel in that sense the outsider. That's perhaps also a spring of why I do what I do which is social art in a sense, social activity, and it's also part of my insecurity about social occasions.

CLARE: An outsider?

HALL: I've always been an outsider and the kind of cliché of those times — working class boy who went to the village school and then to elementary school and then won a scholarship to the grammar school and then won a scholarship to Cambridge. But I still felt that I was the outsider who was arriving, trying to become something he wasn't. To some degree I've always felt the same in the theatre.

CLARE: Trying to become something you weren't?

HALL: Not trying, not so much trying as being put in a situation where you were playing a game by a set of rules which were perhaps not entirely yours. I mean in terms of money and position and all the rest.

CLARE: Would your mother or father talk about any of this? Were you conscious, growing up, that such divisions existed?

HALL: Yes. The greatest tragedy to me of my childhood is that everything that happened to me from about eight years old divided me from my parents. I mean they were not, how could they be, why should they be, very very well educated. They were intelligent people, they were working-class people, they were warm-hearted people, but everything I was interested in, everything that I became, everything that I learnt, made a huge gulf between them and me, and by the time I was in my twenties it was terribly difficult for me to communicate with them and for them to communicate with me. They were inordinately proud and supportive of me but we were like foreigners from different countries and it wasn't until much, much later (and they died a couple of years ago both in the same week) that I appreciated, I think, them and maybe they appreciated me, with the relaxation that comes with old age.

CLARE: Did they worry about you?

HALL: Oh very very much. I mean I was the first person in my family to get to a university, and I was supposed to get a proper job, not go into the theatre. The fact that having come that route and they'd skimped and saved and sacrificed so that I could go on that educational route, the fact that I announced that I was going to go into the theatre alarmed them greatly, and with reason. I mean, I got a first in my first year and a two-one in my second year and a two-two in my third year and if there had been a fourth year I would have failed because I was doing nothing but theatre.

CLARE: Did your mother ever articulate what it was she would like Peter to be? Did she have at the back of her mind something that she saw you as?

HALL: I think she wanted me to be successful whatever that means and well-off and secure, I think the kind of ups and downs, the fever chart of a professional theatre life did give her great anxiety all her years. The fact that I think in many respects my professional life and the pressures of my professional life have been one of the reasons that my private life has been chequered, I think that disturbed her certainly. But they never interfered, they were supportive and I would lay my hand on my heart and say they were model parents in trying to allow me to grow in whatever direction I needed to grow even though it took me away from them.

CLARE: Were you an insufferable adolescent?

HALL: I think I was a difficult adolescent, but then I think everybody is. I don't think I was particularly insufferable. I don't think they over-indulged me, I think their set of rules really was that education could do it but as a corollary of that, hard work could do it. I mean they believed in the East Anglian work ethic which was very strong, the puritan work ethic.

CLARE: But one of the experiences of an only child is he or she is in a sense the centre of attention, they don't have to share it with anybody.

HALL: It was made even worse for me actually, because I was not only the only child of my parents' marriage, I was the only child for about eleven or twelve years of a very large, very tightly inter-related family of uncles and aunts and grandmothers and grandfathers and all that.

CLARE: You mentioned the loneliness of being an only child to which I'm sure we will return, but I was thinking much more of the strange sense of all-importance.

HALL: I think it was much more a sense of high expectation. I was supposed to be a high achiever. I mean my first audience, my first public was the family, and they expected high achievement of me and hard work.

CLARE: Did you ever feel irritated or even angry about such a burden?

HALL: I felt terribly anxious because one of the things about the scholarship route is that you really quite early become aware that if you fail the hurdle the whole course of your life will change. I could not have done what I have done if I hadn't gone to grammar school and if I hadn't gone to

Cambridge. I have no doubt at all about that. You know, I don't know what I would have ended up as doing, can't imagine.

CLARE: So to use the image that you gave me, the jag sequence certainly was present even in the sense that there would be the hurdle which you would approach with considerable anxiety and then overcome it with considerable triumph. This family, this extended family would have, I take it, shared in your triumphs, the scholarship to grammar school was their triumph, going to Cambridge would have been a great triumph? Is that what you recall? Can you recall the day you got the scholarship?

HALL: Yes I remember the letter coming, absolutely, and I remember, you know, not only did I get school prizes as you do, for English or History or whatever, I also got prizes from aunts and uncles for getting the prizes, or for getting the scholarship. I've got quite a number of books written in by members of the family, books that, you know, they would always say to me what would you like, so an early volume of C Day Lewis or Bernard Shaw, and that pattern of putting yourself on the line and being judged, succeeding or not succeeding has gone on right through my life. I mean one of the curious things about my profession is that although you can say you're a doctor or a lawyer, solicitor, an accountant, if you do something not well you'll get a bad reputation, but you are not judged on every single transaction that you do, and your rating is not as good as your last case, that's not quite so in the theatre. You're only as good as your last play to some extent and you are judged in a fierce spotlight.

CLARE: That also illustrates why so frequently people from your world say that phrase 'Some day I've got this feeling I'll be found out.'

HALL: Well I think we all feel that. I certainly feel that. I feel that because, although I know my craft, I'm also aware that being a director who does a good job is as much a subjective or instinctive thing as being a performer or an actor or any other kind of interpretative artist. There are things that you don't know where they come from. If I stand in a rehearsal and think 'My God, what should I do?' In other words I mentally turn up the chapter of the craft, I'm dead. I hear myself saying something, then I'm directing, I do it. And therefore, you know, sometimes the gift is with you and sometimes it isn't. Sometimes if you do something which doesn't work, and the press says 'This is a ghastly production, it's awful, it doesn't work,' you think, 'Well maybe I can't do it.' That's what we all feel in our profession. I think it is nerve-racking but it is also extremely healthy. You can't take refuge in position, you really can't and you can't say 'I've been doing this for thirty-five years, I know how to do it,' because the public and the critics will say 'We don't care how long you've been doing it for, what was this production like?'

CLARE: But combine that reality of the craft with your particular background, psychology and it is potentially exhausting. I am beginning to get a picture of a person who from very early on carried the expectations of large numbers of people, on your own, which is something I do want to talk to you about. All directors will to some extent be doing what you described yourself as doing. They may come from very different backgrounds, but few may be carrying that intensity of need to achieve that you carry.

HALL: What you say I recognise. I not only wanted to be the person who made the play happen, the director, I also wanted to be the person who ran the theatre, who employed the director.

CLARE: The interesting feature of your early life would have been the extent to which you did it all yourself. These parents, they helped, by the way you've described, by their enormous support clearly they provided you with a basket of relationships that sustained you, but nonetheless you did it, you went into the exam, you got the scholarship, you went to Cambridge, and you did this with, as far as I can make out, no one else, really.

HALL: It was solo, certainly and it was certainly solo in terms of near relations or friends. I was blessed with four wonderful schoolmasters. It doesn't matter what school you go to, the thing is did you meet a good teacher? And I had four at various times that I really owe an enormous lot to, and those I remember with real, real gratitude. They fostered my ambitions. They fostered me in every kind of way, and they of course became more important than anybody in the family.

CLARE: What would have been the first time when you had to very obviously or explicitly live in a team situation?

HALL: In a team? I think I did that at school. You see the other thing I discovered, again I don't know why or how, but I discovered it at school, that although I was shy and although I felt awkward people would follow me. I discovered that they would consent to be led by me. I organised things at school and I was head prefect and all that kind of thing so I took on some of the social responsibilities of the school in that sense.

CLARE: When did you realise that you and your parents were separating? How early would it have been that you realised that the experiences you were having were actually taking you away and in one sense giving you abilities and skills and knowledge they didn't have?

HALL: It was around eight or nine. I know that because the kind of music they liked on the whole was operettas, popular music, Gilbert and Sullivan, and I was very quickly moving away from that, and I was very quickly moving away from their kind of books. My tenth birthday I remember, it sounds extremely precocious but I remember it, I asked if I could go to Kings College Chapel, Cambridge, to hear Mozart's Requiem and I did, my mother took me. And the following week I saw *The Marriage of Figaro* for the first time. Sadlers Wells were evacuated to Cambridge, this was 1940.

CLARE: How would you have heard, before you went there?

HALL: Of Mozart?

CLARE: Exactly.

HALL: I was an absolutely voracious reader. I can't remember when I first heard about Mozart. I certainly, by the time I was ten, had played Mozart on the piano but libraries were my joy. Reading was my ordinary way I lived. I read all the time, I read on the bus to school, on the train to school.

CLARE: Do you think that contributed to your confidence as a leader, the fact that very early on, earlier than many children, you realised that you possessed certain skills, knowledge, abilities that gave you in some sense power, influence?

HALL: It could be but as the minor scholar, as the working class scholarship boy I was always somewhat surprised that I was allowed to be the leader. I suppose the most extraordinary thing looking back on it is that when I was nine, eight, nine, my father moved to the outskirts of Cambridge, because he went on the relief as a station master, when anybody was ill or on holiday he would go to the small stations around Cambridgeshire. So suddenly I was in a, for me, big town, and I remember an emotional shock, I remember crying for days because the streets frightened me actually, as we had lived absolutely in the country and I, I still feel that's where my roots are, I don't like town living actually. Anyway, but there was Cambridge from ten or nine on as an absolute feast of music and drama, particularly in the early war years, because of people being evacuated from London. So I saw Gielgud's *Hamlet* when I was twelve. I heard the Mozart that I've just been describing, and because my father had free rail travel and I had an aunt in Lewisham, by the time I was fourteen I was coming up to London, even though it was wartime, and seeing plays, and by the time I was fourteen I wanted to be a director. I didn't quite know what a director was, except I knew that somebody made it happen and it was what I wanted – to make it happen.

CLARE: You say that when you started to mix with other children you were conscious of your powers as a leader, someone who got things going from early on. What would have been your first experiences of relating to the opposite sex?

HALL: Oh very very very difficult, because having had no sisters and having had no girls or young women in the family I mean girls were absolutely foreign creatures to me, by the time one reached the lower-sixth form there were the school dancing classes with the Girls School. I was terribly awkward and shy, I didn't know how to talk to girls in my early or mid teens, certainly not, but in so far as I know myself I am very romantic and very idealistic, and believe very very much in love between the sexes. I wanted to be absolute and the best and one's ability to be disappointed if it's less than the best is very profound.

CLARE: How do those two elements in your character, the idealism and the ability to and a desire to control, to direct, to run things, how do they co-exist?

HALL: I'm not sure whether it's control, so much as to enable. I mean it's not just a judgemental remark, I direct plays, not for the money, the fame, the notices or the audience. If I'm honest, I direct plays because if you have a good piece of material and a good cast in any rehearsal period there are at least two days when the actors are all better than they had a right to expect and you, the director, are better, when something absolutely extraordinary happens to you collectively as a group. That gives me the greatest buzz in the world, that's why I do it.

CLARE: Right, if we say to enable, nonetheless the very title 'director' says that in the end you are in charge. The one area where liking being in charge can provide difficulties is in personal relationships and I wondered how much that made difficulties in your personal life?

HALL: I'm sure it has. There aren't enough hours in the day to pursue what I've been driven to pursue. I'm sure it has, although without wishing to boast, I think that my children have accepted what I am and I feel extraordinarily close to all five of them.

CLARE: When you say your children have accepted what you are, what do you mean?

HALL: That I overwork, and that I don't normally take holidays.

CLARE: You overwork. You don't take holidays. You don't have time for anybody else but you or this craft or this calling. I've talked to others who would speak very similarly. But what about the people who live around them who are in the shadow of this great driving passion. Later, when they grow they understand it, no doubt, but as you said, your children, you're talking about say Jennifer, Christopher, your older children, it would have meant that as they were growing up, you wouldn't have had the time for them that they would have wanted?

HALL: I'm sure that's true, but I'm sure the time, I don't know, I, I hope the time I did give them was a hundred per cent.

CLARE: It almost certainly would be given your character, but wouldn't that only make it all the more difficult, a hundred per cent of your time for a short time would make people want more?

HALL: I would like to live my life again with a thirty-six-hour day, because I love children, and I've loved my children and I do have regrets in this area. I also feel that I've been extraordinarily blessed because I've had over thirty years of small children and I think children from, I don't know, two until nine or ten are the most extraordinary windows on the world. They remind you of all sorts of things that you forget.

CLARE: But Sir Peter there will be people listening, particularly women listening who'll say, that is a typical male observation. I read something about you in your diaries or it was about you somewhere else, that one year you'd six Sundays or something spare for your family. Listeners will say that wretched man, namely me, is going to let Sir Peter off with that romantic observation about small children, but he would have hardly seen them as small children!

HALL: This is a very hard question. If you are engaged in a profession which is obsessional, which is not simply to pass the time, not simply to earn the money, but which is actually obsessional, which gives you the greatest joy and the greatest fulfilment, there are distortions I'm sure, but you can't actually do anything about it, because you are blessed or cursed with that obsession. I mean it's absolutely no good me saying to myself I will work less hard. Christopher, when he was about ten said to me 'Why do you work so hard Papa? What are you trying to prove?,' which I thought was an extraordinarily acute observation. And I said I'm not trying to prove anything, I like it, I actually like it.

CLARE: Then let me put a different question. Is what we are talking about not just an obsession but a sort of time greed? You said 'I wish it was a thirty-six hour day.' You're greedy for the time. You eat it up in a sense.

HALL: Yes, I love just catching trains. I love fitting in more than is possible in one day.

CLARE: You dislike periods when nothing much happens?

HALL: Oh I can't bear them, simply can't bear them. I mean, all right my idea of a holiday is something that has to be prepared or written or achieved in congenial surroundings. But to do nothing, to unwind, to relax I don't understand those things at all, because I don't need to do it, I don't feel the need to do it in that sense.

CLARE: Are you a man with great appetites?

HALL: Yes.

CLARE: Food?

HALL: Yes.

CLARE: Alcohol?

HALL: No.

CLARE: Sex?

HALL: Yes.

CLARE: You recognise that about yourself?

HALL: Oh, yes. I haven't a great appetite for alcohol because I simply loathe losing control. I loathe, you know, actually not being in command of my faculties, that's why I don't much like alcohol.

CLARE: So it might be better if we saw your drive not so much as obsession but more as greed. Obsession suggests that it drives you and there's an element of resistance on your part, that you would prefer that it were not so.

HALL: Oh, no, I don't. I think the element of competitiveness is important. I am greedy to do it, but I don't think it's a race which I've got to win, do you understand what I mean? I mean I don't do a great deal more work than most of my colleagues because I want to stop them doing work or get ahead of the game, I've also had thirty years of employing my colleagues and that's been a very treasured experience, I really have loved that, being a producer.

CLARE: Where the word 'obsession' however may be fair enough, or 'compulsive' might even be better, is the extent to which you say you couldn't actually not do this, you could not actually slow down or fit less into the twenty-four hours rather than looking for thirty-six.

HALL: I think I'm better at it now as I approach sixty than I was when I was thirty. Because I know myself I think well enough now to not overstep the mark, but I want to be on the mark all the time. I certainly don't want to go slower, I certainly don't want to do less, I've certainly no idea of retiring. I couldn't even contemplate the thought.

CLARE: If your son had said to you 'Papa,' instead of saying, 'What are you trying to prove?' if he'd said 'Is there something you're afraid of?'

HALL: Well the thing I'm afraid of is that I won't have a job, I won't be able to do this thing which delights me so much. It really does delight me.

CLARE: Have there been periods in your life of enforced idleness or periods when you were just not able to do anything very much?

HALL: No, there was three weeks when I was in the RAF when they couldn't decide whether to post me to Germany or the Far East and they put me in one of those transit camps and there was nothing to do all day except go to the Naffi and eat your buns and that's the only time I can think of. I read *War and Peace*. I set myself a big task that, you know, this was the time to do it. You see, I'm ashamed to say this in this profession because of the deprivation that so many people have in it, I have never been out of work but one of the reasons for that is that I always arrange so many things to do.

CLARE: Has it ever got to the stage where it has almost destroyed you?

HALL: Yes, once, in the early years of the RSC. We'd just moved to the Aldwych, I'd just started the whole thing going. My first marriage was rocky.

CLARE: That was to Leslie Caron, the actress . . .

HALL: Yes, I had not yet made the Royal Shakespeare Company. I was in the process of trying to prove the point. I set about doing the Henry VI plays which we called *The Wars of The Roses* which was a huge epic undertaking of four plays and something I'd wanted to do all my life and I very nearly, well I did crack up. I rehearsed for about ten days and collapsed and the doctor said, 'Six months rest, you're just totally fatigued.' So I was put to bed and there was great debate about whether the production should be cancelled and whatever. It was Peter Brook and Peggy Ashcroft, close friends, Peggy was in the production, who came and talked to me and said 'Come back and do it now, just as soon as you can.' So I was off for a fortnight and then I went back and did it. I was terribly tired and terribly miserable and actually didn't enjoy doing it but I think it's probably the best thing I've ever done. That's another paradox!

CLARE: How depressed did you get?

HALL: Terribly. I mean illogical, irrational . . .

CLARE: To the point of feeling that you could not go on?

HALL: Yes. Yes.

CLARE: Has that happened to you since?

HALL: Not, no, not to the same extent. I say not to the same extent, because I have I think a tendency at the end of each day to slump, after all this hyperactivity, my most depressive moments are just before I go to sleep, always. I suppose that's when the adrenalin drops.

CLARE: And you feel low?

HALL: And I feel low, yes.

CLARE: And doubt? Whether the effort has been worth it?

HALL: Yes, but the next morning there's the joy of going back to it again. I can't imagine not doing it.

CLARE: Your first marriage broke up, to some extent, over this very issue.

HALL: Yes, we were two professional people in highly successful positions and the demands on each of us were different geographically and in every other respect.

CLARE: The reference I saw suggested that she felt, Leslie Caron felt, that you didn't need to do this amount of work, that it was actually under your control, that you were actually choosing to work this extraordinary routine.

HALL: I think that's a point of view. I mean I don't actually believe it myself but I can see why she would.

CLARE: It never disturbed you. You never said to yourself 'This is a compulsion to work.' You saw how other people work. In general your work rate is pretty phenomenal.

HALL: Yes, except I know plenty of people who write music or write plays or write books like water coming out of a tap, because they're born to do it. Now it would be presumptuous of me to say I'm born to do this but I don't know any other way of living. I try not to hurt the people around me or deprive the people around me by so doing, but it is what I am and it's difficult not to be what I am and you know as far as all the marriages are concerned it may sound paradoxical for somebody who's been divorced three times to say I believe passionately in marriage, but I do.

CLARE: Why?

HALL: Because I believe that an absolute sharing with someone you love of all you believe in and all you do, a complete open sharing allied to the physical and emotional union is about the greatest thing I know, and hard to achieve.

CLARE: For someone to do it with you, she would have to understand this crucial element in your character, the compulsion to work.

HALL: Yes.

CLARE: I was struck by the fact that your second marriage which lasted very much longer was to someone who knew the business. Jacqueline Taylor had been your secretary and in that sense she understood the way you were?

HALL: Yes, I think she was also very responsive and committed to the children, both my first lot of children and the children we had together. I'm sure that living with me means sacrifices. I'm sure that I try to make sacrifices but I can't not be what I have to be. I wouldn't expect a woman to be any different. I have been married to two great artistes, great artistes, Leslie Caron, and Maria Ewing who was, I think, one of the greatest opera singers I've ever seen. Their compulsions professionally are not very different from mine, they can't be because it is that need to express, and that need to do what you need to do in order to express. It's very hard to have a twin course though with two people like that.

CLARE: It's actually impossible?

HALL: I don't know whether it's impossible. That would be presumptuous, I wouldn't say that. I don't know whether I've ever seen two careers blossom together. Now is that because of the social pressure of marriage or is it because somebody has to be the boss? I don't know.

CLARE: But doesn't a relationship ultimately depend on the extent to which there's time?

HALL: Oh yes certainly, but . . .

CLARE: But your time is . . .

HALL: . . . I've had . . .

CLARE: . . . terribly fully committed.

HALL: Yes but, you know I think one has to get it in proportion. My observation of most people is that they're lazy and that they waste time, and that one of their satisfactions is to waste time. My satisfaction is not to waste time. Although I'm sitting in your chair or lying on your couch metaphorically, I find it difficult and almost undesirable to talk about the complexities of my failed marriages, because so much of each of them were so good and when you start talking about the failure you emphasise the negative, and certainly you start feeling your own responsibilities to those failures. But I have, for the last two years, been with another lady, Nicky Fry, who I'm going to marry for the fourth try, and I've been happier than I have ever been. It would require very complex analysis to find out why that's working and you might say well it's not going to go on working, none of the others have. I don't know, but I have hope. And certainly time is necessary, but you can make time.

CLARE: I'm struck that you never seem to have said, after one or other of these relationships came to a painful ending, as some do, enough is enough, I need time. You've actually moved very quickly. You're a man who needs marriage?

HALL: Yes I do.

CLARE: What is it that you need?

HALL: Well, it's companionship, it's love, it's understanding, it's actually just also having somebody that you can tell everything to. I mean I'm not saying every marriage allows that, but that would be my definition of marriage.

CLARE: So despite having grown up an only child, you're not someone who really can live an isolated life?

HALL: I don't like being alone.

CLARE: How do you think you would be if you weren't married? What sort of person would you be on your own?

HALL: I think I would be tenser, probably more inclined to paranoia, probably more uncertain, and frustrated, both emotionally and sexually.

CLARE: Paranoia is a word that crops up frequently in the diaries.

HALL: Yes it is because you know if you're also in public life you get attacked all the time. It goes with being in public life. It's very hard to remind yourself that it is not primarily because of you but because you are standing in the position in which you are standing. There are always certain drama critics that you know who don't like you for whatever reason and they'll never like anything you do. And since anything you do has good and bad in it, whether a critic is disposed to look for the good or emphasise the bad is to do with his prejudice. I'm not saying he shouldn't have it, but you know you've got to be very very careful about that. And then if you're running something like the National Theatre which if it's fulfilling its position in the country is a kind of Aunt Sally for every pressure group and every loony in the land, you find that you're often seen to be doing something wrong.

CLARE: How did you cope?

HALL: I think I could best describe it by metaphor, by taking the fall and then getting straight up again and going, getting on. I mean you cannot develop a thick skin, you cannot say it's not happening, you can't pretend that you're not getting abused and criticised and refuse to read it, I mean that's defensive. You have to go with it, suffer and get straight up and go on and that's hard, but I try to train myself to do that.

CLARE: Is this sometimes seen as insensitivity?

HALL: Yes, I think some people think that I am terribly thick-skinned and terribly arrogant and terribly self-contained, and not at all easily hurt.

CLARE: Because that's to some extent the front you've put on.

HALL: Yes that's my mask.

CLARE: So what do they make of an entry in your diary, 'I have been thrashing with the desperation of the insecure for twenty-five years and I am no nearer making it now than when I came out of Cambridge because one never really makes it'?

HALL: The greatest people I know who you would think have got everything are desperately insecure. Laurence Olivier had chronic stage fright. I've watched him having it for seven or eight years in his late fifties and early sixties. Stage fright? Olivier? He could hardly get on the stage. The greatest artists believe when they've finished writing something they'll never write again. I'm not putting myself in that kind of class. I'm an interpretative man. But when I've done a good piece of work I have two or three hours of satisfaction or dissatisfaction and then it all has to be done again. I think the important lesson is that that kind of insecurity is not something special to you, it's the human condition and you have just got to learn to deal with it.

CLARE: But one of the ways that you deal with it suggests to other people that you're not insecure at all, that you're arrogant, confident, difficult?

HALL: Oh, yes. Well I'm very difficult because I believe what I believe, and I know that if you compromise on your beliefs for whatever reason in my particular field, you have absolutely nothing at all left, nothing. It's important in any job that I do that I can leave it, because if I am asked to do things which seem to me against what I believe then I must be able to go, and I've always felt that, crucially. I'm difficult because I'm very demanding. I think I am a perfectionist in my work and I expect everybody else to have the same kind of input. Some people like that, and some people don't. I mean I have the greatest respect for the creativity of the actor or of any of the people who're working with me, the designers, the composers or whatever, and a director's job is not to tell everybody what to do, a director's job is to bring the best out of everybody and make them do something that surprises even them. I directed Laurence Olivier when I was twenty-six, twenty-seven and people said to me, 'How on earth do you tell Lawrence Olivier what to do?' I said, 'You don't tell him what to do. That's not what a director is. A director is there to suggest and provoke and be a mirror for the actor and then finally an editor.'

CLARE: Being a director – it is a manipulative skill?

HALL: Yes, certainly it is a manipulative skill.

CLARE: So in that sense you are a manipulative person.

HALL: Any director is a manipulative person. Not only are you manipulative, you have a different persona to some extent, a different mask to everybody you deal with.

CLARE: Are you conscious of those skills in general, that you have an ability to get round people, if you want to?

HALL: Yes, that's why I like committees!

CLARE: You do?

HALL: Yes, and I like, if I win, yes, I like politics in that sense.

CLARE: So you can be charming, tough, bullying, seductive, and you would know you were doing it?

HALL: I always know I'm doing it.

CLARE: So there's an element of being detached as you do it.

HALL: Yes, because the real me is none of those things and is actually quite shy as I said.

CLARE: Can I push you a little about it, because the real you you say is shy, but the real you is also those things we've just described, isn't it? I mean they are abilities that you have and have to a fairly well-developed extent.

HALL: Certainly I get a very good adrenalin buzz out of a board meeting or a meeting with the Arts Council, I did in the old days when I was running the RSC and the National. And I get the same sort of buzz out of a good rehearsal or out of giving a public lecture. But after it there's always a feeling of letdown, of some despair, the reality behind the mask. But, I mean, I don't know to what extent everybody feels that, because any form of social behaviour is putting on a mask. I mean if you sit alone in a room and someone knocks at the door, as the knock happens something happens to you, the way you look, the way you present yourself, no matter who comes in, one better not think oneself too special for that. Manipulating people is a charge that is always levied at directors, but it can be the same kind of soft cliché as saying that an actor is always impersonating somebody else, so he doesn't finally know who he is. Manipulation to me has the sense that there will be an imminent crack of the bone as it's forced. My manipulation in rehearsal is not by force, can't be, it's by consent.

CLARE: Your parents died in 1988 within a week of each other, I believe. You had come closer again.

HALL: They came to live right next door to us in Oxfordshire in Wallingford where we were living and therefore one saw more of them and they had the grandchildren. I think they relaxed and I relaxed and I came to value particularly my father's tolerance and, and understanding that there are no final battles to be won.

CLARE: His tolerance in relation to you would have been displayed in what sort of circumstances?

HALL: Well he was terribly interested in all the political side of my life and he was a staunch Trade Unionist and was terribly interested in all the Labour troubles we had.

CLARE: What did he make of the fact that you couldn't be, I think, described as a staunch Socialist?

HALL: Well I think he thought I could be. I've only voted Conservative once in my life, and that was in 1979 when I thought that the Conservative Party and Thatcher was about the only hope of stopping an undemocratic power base in the unions wrecking everything I liked about this country, and I don't regret that, because she did. She then proceeded, as far as I'm concerned, to wreck our education system and our broadcasting and our performing arts, and those are things I care passionately about, so I'm very hostile to the legacy this government is leaving. As far as my father was concerned I was brought up Labour and a union man. I remember his jubilation when the railways were national-ised, but I also remember his disillusionment when nation-alisation had produced uniformity and inefficiency and dirty carriages and late trains. He was of the generation of brass watches and shiny carriages and all that, you know, well-kept stations, very different world. When I said to him, I used to go down on Sundays to see them, and I said 'We have an unofficial strike at the National Theatre but the union have said that the picket is official,' my father said, 'It can't possibly be an official picket with unofficial strikers, sack the lot of them. The union is bringing the whole movement into disrepute.' So I had to explain to him that we were living in slightly different times. But he loved all that. He was very interested in politics and I'm sure I get a lot of that from him. My mother wasn't.

CLARE: What did they make of your knighthood?

HALL: Oh they were absolutely thrilled. I'll tell you a funny story. For some curious reason, the letter informing me that should I accept it I might be offered a knighthood was sent by some mistake to my parents' house and my father phoned me up and said, 'There's a very official letter here,' he said, 'I'm afraid it's from the police.' He said, 'What have you been doing?' and he then opened it and read and was overjoyed, it was very nice.

CLARE: Did you have any doubts about being Sir Peter Hall?

HALL: Yes I was terribly worried that I would cease to be a working director and that people in the rehearsal room would start treating me as some kind of totem to be mocked, abused or respected. Any of those things would be dreadful. I've finally resolved that it was offered in a good spirit as a recognition of what I'd been trying to do, and one must accept it graciously and in a good spirit.

CLARE: The reason I ask is something you said earlier. You said, it's a very striking image, 'We all wear masks to some extent.' You say, we sit in a room, somebody knocks on the door and instantly various things change. I wonder whether you're saying there were no perceptible changes in you, once this had happened to you? Though in fact of course the moment you're called Sir Peter Hall all sorts of small, perhaps largely insignificant things happen.

HALL: Bills tend to get larger!

CLARE: There are more significant things I suppose?

HALL: I'll tell you. The new mask that I've adopted is not being a knight. I mean I will not be called Sir Peter in any organisation that I run or in any rehearsal that I conduct. I'm Peter, so you can say that I'm kind of inverting the whole thing and trading on it. I suppose to some degree that could be true.

CLARE: And you've done that because you've seen what happens in terms of other people being knighted?

HALL: I've seen a certain reverential pomposity develop and young actors either, you know, thinking that they won't talk openly in rehearsal because the man is either kind of elevated and on high or because he's ridiculous because he's now a kind of establishment figure. Either way, as I say, is contrary to the work process. I must confess that being knighted for the Royal Shakespeare Company and the National Theatre gave me enormous pleasure and is a little, tiny tiny tiny nugget of security in an insecure world.

CLARE: Is there anything, any achievement, any possession, any external signal, anything that would give you profound security?

HALL: There's no position or recognition, no. I would like to have a home which I love and which is mine and I could stay in for the rest of my life, that I would like. That I don't have, because of the complexities of my life, the pressure of my life and the fact that I've actually never made any money. I've always lived well within the province of my professional pressure. I have enough money to finance the way I live, but I have no savings, no pension, no security and if I'm unable to work tomorrow I wouldn't have any resources. I haven't made any money because I've chosen not to. I've always done what I wanted to do artistically and sometimes that brings in money and sometimes it doesn't, and in my case it hasn't on the whole. But I would like a place in the country and I stress country, but that's probably you know like everybody's dream of a country cottage with roses – it's probably just a fantasy.

CLARE: Do you think about death?

HALL: Oh, yes, every day. I don't think you can shut that out.

CLARE: What aspect of it?

HALL: Well it frightens me very much because I do believe that it's extinction.

CLARE: There's nothing afterwards.

HALL: That's what I believe and I find, as everybody does, that a very difficult thought to come to terms with. I don't know how well I shall cope with pain, suffering, the kind of pain and suffering I saw my mother go through, the awful rage she developed against it which I can well understand, I don't know how, how courageous I would be in that. I would like to die without many regrets. It's very interesting, you see, if you exercise power and you exercise choice and you do, as you've said, to some degree manipulate or order other people's lives, people begin to give you motives which are often evil and irresponsible. I can best illustrate it anyway by saying that however great the actor, the moment he comes to be directed by me or by anybody else he puts his talent in the palm of your hand like an egg and the temptation to squeeze it is horrible but there, and you mustn't, obviously you mustn't.

CLARE: Have you ever done it?

HALL: No, I don't think so. Perhaps there's some actor listening who'll say I have, but I fervently believe that I've never done it, but I'm very aware of it.

CLARE: You've seen it done.

HALL: I've seen it done. I have indeed seen it done many times. I don't like manipulation when it's evil, I don't like sadism. I believe in tolerance and I believe in compassion, and I believe in freedom of speech and freedom of expression. I hate censorship, I hate do-gooders, I hate people who tell me or anybody else what they ought to believe or what they ought to do. The human spirit is free and must be allowed to be free, always with the proviso that we cannot hurt other people. We must understand that. those are the clichés I believe in. They're hard to live by and they're hard to work by, but in a way my work is at the sharp end of all that, which is why I like it, I cannot afford to be insensitive because if I am I won't work. No actor will work with me. I cannot afford to be stupid or inconsiderate or just out for myself because people will not work with me either, that's what's good about my profession. I think I'm better at it now than I was thirty-five years ago. I think I'm as good now as I've ever been but I still want to get better. I want to have an Indian summer of being a director, and I hope my health and strength will allow me to because I love it. I don't think I shall ever be prepared for death. You can't tell but I suppose the people who are prepared for death have a really understanding recognition that life is over and that pain can't go on. My father was prepared for death. My mother was in hospital in a coma and I was asked to tell my father that she was not going to recover. And I said to him 'You know mother's not going to come home, she's going to die in the next ten days or so.' And he said 'Yes I know.' And I said 'Well you know you must come and live with me in London while we sort everything out.' He said 'Let's talk about that when she's gone, and I'll see you on Sunday.' So I went back to London and on the Saturday morning I rang him to make the arrangements for going down on Sunday and taking him out to lunch and he was fine, and he had his lunch on Saturday and took his nap after lunch which he always did and died. So he never knew that mother had died and mother never knew that he had died, and my mother died on his funeral day, when I buried him. He was eighty-six years old, he'd decided that was enough and it was sort of beautiful actually and he was blessed to go like that I suppose. I dread pain and fury and suffering.

CLARE: It's a good life you've had?

HALL: I've had a very good life, I actually have no complaints. I have been blessed to have an obsession and the world has allowed me to do it. I know lots of people who have obsessions and they're not allowed to exercise them. I'm very lucky. I have five wonderful children. I have a lot of wonderful friends and I've had, although a bumpy private life, a wonderful private life. I am actually happier now than I've ever been in my life, I have to say that though hubris makes me a little nervous about saying it.

Anthony Hopkins

When in 1982 I was being interviewed for the Chair of Psychological Medicine at St Bartholomew's Hospital Medical College, a member of the appointments committee, the late and much lamented Professor Kenneth Rawnsley, a former President of the Royal College of Psychiatrists and then Head of the Academic Department of Psychological Medicine at Cardiff, queried the title of *In the Psychiatrist's Chair* (the series had just started) on the grounds that what happens in the interviews is not psychiatric, the subjects are not patients and there is no treatment. The points are reasonable. Indeed, Rawnsley's objections had been anticipated at the time the title was chosen. However, Michael Ember, the producer, felt, rightly I believe, that some explicit reference had to be made to the fact that I was a psychiatrist and a title that did that would also make explicit the point of the interviews, namely that the focus would be on the early experiences, the drives, the motives, the stresses and strains characterising the lives of interviewees. No sensible person, participant or listener, surely would presume that a half hour interview with anybody could amount to therapy (although several interviewees have been kind enough to say they felt better after the exchange! Nobody as far as I know felt worse). Nor does anybody acquire or manifest the status of patient. I am a psychiatrist and it is my chair. To that extent the title makes sense.

But every now and again somone does sit in it and behave just like someone would in a therapeutic situation. Anthony Hopkins certainly did. He is a man who has been through dark times. He speaks of the role played by that remarkable support group, the forerunner of all the voluntary self-help organis- ations around the world, namely Alcoholics Anonymous, in helping him back to sanity and stability. He is still preoccupied with making sense of who and what he is and he is open enough to admit to all sorts of doubts and fears. While no longer what he was once termed 'a bundle of sweating Welsh neurosis' he still struggles to make sense of his life and understand what it is all about.

In this interview he insists that acting for him has been a form of therapy, a process which has enabled him to exorcise the anger, frustration, self-doubt which he traces back to his childhood. The way he acts is instinctive rather than methodical. He has to generate a vision of the character he is to play. He gives the examples of Hannibal Lecter in *The Silence of the Lambs*, Dafyd Ap Llewellyn in *A Chorus of Disapproval*, Lambert le Roux in *Pravda*, Henry Wilcox in *Howards End*. A gifted mimic, he draws on this skill and a remarkable memory in which he has stored all sorts of bits and pieces of personalities he had known to build a plausible, convincing, authentic, believable character. Characters that demand a different approach, that require him to construct some internal, psychological model, that do not lend themselves to being constructed from without, Shakespearean characters such as Lear or Pericles, for example, pose problems. He, who is absorbed by the problem of what makes himself tick, is not greatly interested in the motivations of the characters he is asked to play. Intuitively drawn to playing characters who illuminate the dark side of human nature, he explains this by reference to the turbulent, aggressive, unpleasant side of his own character which was so often manifest when he was drinking heavily and profoundly dissatisfied with himself and his life. There is much that is intriguing about him as a man and actor, nothing more than the question he raises about one's ability to act oneself into a state of mind, a conviction of oneself. In the interview he describes how he tells friends who are feeling depressed, 'Well act as if you're happy.' When his wife suggests that, being Welsh, he is bound to experience melancholic swings that is a cue for him to kick the part and choose another. The little boy from Port Talbot who hadn't a clue who he was, who felt as if he should have been on another planet, whose baffled and disapproving father wondered what would become of him, has become all sorts of people by virtue of his extraordinary talent as an actor – so why not play the part of being happy even when you're not, indeed especially when you are not?

As he told it to me, it did appear to be working. There were of course other factors operating as he is the first to admit, the triumph of *The Silence of the Lambs* being just one of them. Nevertheless, thinking positively has helped him. Some, particularly psychotherapists of a classical psychoanalytic persuasion, would be concerned about the possibility of self-delusion, about the possibility that Hopkins has just chosen to play yet another role, that of the contented, recovered alcoholic, and that he is no nearer finding out who he really is while he buries himself in a succession of somebody elses. Yet there are echoes in his approach of a form of psychotherapy which has recently become popular, namely cognitive therapy.

At the heart of the therapy is a recognition of the fact that depressed people tend to think negatively about life, tend to over-generalise from a few bad things happening to the conclusion that everything is bleak and irredeemable, tend to magnify setbacks and minimise achievement, tend to notice the flaws, particularly in themselves, and ignore or deny the virtues. This cognitive process acts like a vicious circle, making the depressed person feel even more depressed. Cognitive therapy aims to counter these negative thoughts or cognitions by training the patient to recognise the negative and destructive way he or she automatically responds to everyday stresses and setbacks and the way this amplifies his or her feelings of worthlessness. Various techniques are used, tasks are developed to enable the depressed individual to test and challenge depressing ideas. The sufferer may be encouraged to keep a diary of thoughts and moods with the aim of identifying the repetitive, intrusive thoughts which help to maintain and worsen depressed moods. Common negative thoughts include 'I am of little use to anyone', 'I am never going to feel any different', 'I will never amount to much so I might as well not bother trying'.

In his adolescence Anthony Hopkins remembers getting the feeling that people were saying of him, 'Oh Hopkins, you know, he's well, he's not worth much or he's a failure.' His father, himself a sufferer from melancholic mood swings, a man of fierce discontent and gloomy passion, would hassle and belittle him. As for selective bias for the bad and ignoring the good, it describes most accurately Hopkins's handling of criticism. One smell of failure, one questionable review would unnerve and shake him despite plenty to the contrary. When he felt such failure he would equate it with some moral deficiency in himself. His belief that he was intrinsically worthless was solidly reinforced.

It is clear from what happened to him after adolescence and during his drinking and destructive period that he had incorporated a perniciously negative view of himself within himself. Corrosive self-doubt itself acts as a potent stimulus to drink. And what did alcohol do for Anthony Hopkins? It made him feel like Humphrey Bogart, John Wayne, It made him feel like he belonged. However, the problem with alcohol used as a medicine in this way is that its effects are short-lived and more and more has to be drunk to bring about the original effect. And then the trouble really starts. Alcohol inhibits inhibitions and, in the early stages of its use, it appears to act as a stimulant. In reality it is a potent depressant. Hopkins's natural tendency to depression was aggravated by alcohol. He could not convince himself that acting, at which he clearly excelled – he was the outstanding student of his period at RADA – was important. People who have little faith in themselves commonly denigrate that which they are good at – another negative cognition at work. Hopkins reminded me of a patient of mine, a brilliant university student who got a double first but who was so riddled with self-doubt she concluded that obviously university academic standards were not all they were cracked up to be!

Now, Hopkins has adopted his own cognitive therapeutic approach. He finds it works. He has also been able to forgive his father who, he seems to suggest, transferred unwittingly some of his own personal doubts to his son. Hopkins senior is described as a Willie Loman figure, who, in his son's phrase, 'always believed that he would fail' – the most powerful negative conviction of them all. All these years later it seems reasonable to suggest that much of Anthony Hopkins's discontent owed a great deal to unresolved tensions between the two of them and it certainly makes sense to Hopkins. Being able to forgive – a key marker of recovery from neurotic anger, frustration, despair – has helped him move from a morbidly introspective, temperamental cast of mind to a more positive though still introspective state.

These days he remains curious about what makes him tick when once he was desperate about being alive. Once he was overwhelmed by the process of living, now it fascinates him. 'I am what I am' declares Hopkins and he appears to be able to cope with the implications. There will be those, however, who will say, 'It's all very well for him. He was able to overcome the corrosive doubts and despair of the early years because he had a talent and it has carried him to the pinnacle of a career, to public recognition, to an Oscar. Lucky him, he has been able to challenge his internal doubts with external achievements. The rest of us aren't so lucky.' After all, Jonathan Swift, in the final dark, dismal, illness-ridden years of his life also declared 'I am what I am' but what he was was miserable, dying and alone.

What needs to be remembered, and it may not be clear from this interview, is that Anthony Hopkins began to turn his life around as far back as 1975, over a decade before Hannibal Lecter. Why he stopped drinking and thinking the way he did remains as complicated as why he started in the first place. He does provide clues. His wife had had enough – not for many alcoholics a reason to stop drinking but for those who would prefer to lose the bottle than the wife it can be. On its own it might not have been enough for Hopkins but in addition he had a fright, a near-miss, he could have killed somebody. He started to worry too that alcohol was going to kill him. After all it had killed others including his schooldays' idol, Richard Burton.

Anthony Hopkins reminds us that people in trouble with alcohol are not all in the gutter or in prison or in hospital. Many, perhaps most, are apparently functioning, coping with their hidden addiction while their colleagues in business, industry, the professions, the church, the golf club, the housing estate know little or nothing of what is going on or, as happened in Hopkins's case, do know but feel relatively powerless or disinclined to do anything about it. Many alcoholics, Hopkins points out, are 'successful in acting or the arts or whatever they're doing and they don't see that the world is falling apart around them'.

At the time of writing, his own life is very much together. He has reached some *modus vivendi* with himself yet he is too wise to believe that his troubles are over. Indeed he acknowledges an anxiety that all of this may be an illusion, yet another superb piece of acting which has convinced not merely an audience but the actor himself. Borrowing from the AA philosophy, I would hazard a guess that as long as he notes the pin prick of anxiety about returning to the bad old days the bad old days won't return. We are what we are and that includes our past but we don't need to be imprisoned by it, is Hopkins's message. We can break free.

CLARE: Anthony Hopkins was born in Port Talbot on 31st December 1937. His father was a baker and Anthony was an only child, hopeless at school and good only at piano playing. On leaving school he applied for and won a scholarship to Cardiff College of Music and Drama where he spent two years. Later after National Service he was accepted for RADA and graduated in 1963. He has since become a stage and screen actor of international repute. In 1987 he was awarded the CBE and in 1988 Doctor of Letters at the University of Wales. Anthony Hopkins has been married twice, has one daughter, Abigail, and his most recent screen performance has been that of the homicidal psychiatrist Dr Hannibal Lecter in *The Silence of the Lambs*. Tony Hopkins, why did you agree to this interview?

HOPKINS: Well I get a chance to talk about myself for an hour or so. I've been more interested in the last ten or fifteen years in the workings of the human mind and in my own processes of living and development. This answer really is quite spontaneous because I didn't think you were going to ask me that question but that really is the answer. I've always been a very self-obsessed person as all actors are. I'm fascinated by the workings of the mind and especially of my own place in the universe and my own life development.

CLARE: Were you always self-obsessed?

HOPKINS: Yes, yes ever since I went to school and at about the age of four realised that I was on the wrong planet somehow. I simply didn't belong anywhere, didn't understand any of the other children, my class mates you know, boys, girls, felt very alien and isolated, principally because I was very very slow and backward at school. It was double-Dutch to me. I didn't know what they were talking about. I didn't know what I was doing there. Then I was aware that this caused a problem with my father because he was naturally very worried, as I would be for my own daughter, as any parent would be, my father tended to over-worry a little I suppose.

CLARE: There would have been reports coming back about how you were doing or not doing?

HOPKINS: Yes, and about my general listlessness as a child. I was very slow and introverted, didn't bother with other children, used to stand the other end of the street playing ball on my own, while the other kids were down the other side of the street. I got this sense that there was something odd about me. Looking back over the years, over almost fifty years, it is fifty years now, looking back over those years I don't regret any of it because it was the sort of rocket fuel for me to prove to myself that I wasn't worthless or ill-fitting. It's taken me all of my life to get to this feeling now which has been with me for the last two years and I feel free now of all that, all those demons and ghosts.

CLARE: You use the word 'worthless.' Was that something you would have picked up at home as well?

HOPKINS: Not at home no, my parents were loving, doting parents, perhaps they were a little over-concerned. I was the only child after all. My father died ten years ago. That had quite an impact on my life really. My reaction to my own situation in life was one of deep introspection, although I didn't think I had the mental equipment to be introspective, and that stayed with me for many many years. It's only in recent years that I've become much more, I suppose the word is 'extrovert,' and much more open and certainly much more at peace with myself than I've ever been. I don't understand the process but it is certainly a relief to have come through all that. That feeling of unworthiness or worthlessness has I think by and large left me now. It's like some sort of destiny in me that kept guiding me all through this part of my life. I don't understand any of it. I don't quite grasp at why I, for example, am sitting at this table talking about it because all the laws of logic should put me back in, I don't know, our little house in some part of the world. I don't know what I'd be. I can't second-guess what would have happened to me.

CLARE: Did your parents have any ambition for you? Did they see you as anything in particular as you were growing up?

HOPKINS: I started playing the piano when I was about five, six years of age, and I had a sort of talent, but I am certainly not a skilled pianist now, although I play a lot. I remember my mother's one moment of hope when I went off to piano practice, my first lesson and she had high hopes. My father was a cynic. My father had a favourite cartoon which used to crease him up with laughter, it was a cartoon in that old magazine called *Everybody's*, and I can remember it to this day. There's a photograph of a mother and a father sitting in a chair and this little boy very much like Lord Fauntleroy with a little collar playing a violin and there were two thought clouds, two thought bubbles. There's the mother thinking of her son playing in the Albert Hall and there was his father sitting there thinking of the son playing in the gutter years later, and it made my father laugh so much because he was very realistic about life. My mother like, I suppose, all women was much more visionary, much more optimistic about life, so she always had some faith in me that I was going to be special. But in a way all that feedback, all that information I was getting unsolicited was making me feel that I was somehow special because I remember a rather crucial moment in my life when I was sixteen, going through all the pains of adolescence, and suffering very badly at school from appalling academic reports and dreading the school holidays when the reports would come, and there was the usual gnashing of teeth and frettings and all that and I was standing in the kitchen and they were in the other room and I think we were all about to have a row, the three of us, because my father was very worried. I remember he said to my mother, he said 'There's something wrong with this boy,' and I blazed out, I said, 'One day I'll show you all I am different, I am different and I'm going to be different.' I knew I had some kind of artistic creative streak and I didn't know where it was and I remember I said it with such blazing anger like Jimmy Porter. I said 'One day I'll show you, one day I will prove that I'm not a misfit or that I'm not what you think I am.'

CLARE: Were you a very passionate person as a child, an adolescent?

HOPKINS: I was very bad-tempered. I had terrible rages. I was very emotional. I used to play the piano and I used to weep when I played the piano and I used to listen to music, music had a tremendous effect on me and I used to cry a lot. I used to weep and I used to get terribly moved and I'd live in this fantasy world and I'd go for long walks. I was born in a rather pretty part of Port Talbot. The town was Margham and I know all that area so well and I used to go for long walks and I used to hang about Margham Abbey and the churchyards. I was terribly terribly morbid.

CLARE: What about girls?

HOPKINS: Didn't come into contact with girls until I went to college, Cardiff College of Music and Drama and I was seventeen then and I had never spoken to a girl before. I was very shy. I met my first girlfriend there in fact, she later became an actress. I was always a little wary there, very very fearful of rejection and so never could make a pass at a girl or ask her for a date or anything like that. I was terribly nervous in that area.

CLARE: Was this sense of you being different, was it reinforced by your peers, your contemporaries feeling you were different? Did they treat you as different?

HOPKINS: Well, yes it was pretty obvious to me that I was different. I know this probably sounds a bit paranoid but I think children can be very cruel especially in adolescence, and if you are slow and I was (I was in a school which was quite competitive) and if you are slow you do get a lot of slamming about from other kids. I don't know about girls but I know that boys are very cruel and very tough. It built up a tremendous resentment in me because I was also bad at sport and athletics and all I could do was play the piano. So I always got that sense in my adolescent years that 'Oh, Hopkins, you know he's, well he's not worth much, or he's a failure.' That wasn't just something I projected. That was a fact of my adolescent life. I heard those real voices from outside. They weren't from inside me and the funny thing is they stayed with me for a long long long time until fairly recently. They haunted me and I longed all my life to do one thing and that was to be a big hit in a big play or a hit movie or whatever, childish as it sounds. And this film *Silence of the Lambs* has done it. The oddest thing is that I feel now 'Well that's that, I've done it,' and it's let me out of the cage in a way, metaphorically. It's freed me up. The rest for me is fun. I realised only something just recently the other day I was being interviewed by somebody. They were doing a profile on me. I was having a preliminary interview with these two people and they said, 'Well you seem to take your work very lightly now. Has there been a change in your life?' I said 'Well, yes.' I said 'I don't understand really why this has changed or where this change took place, but I've lost the intensity and I've lost the drive to score and it is the oddest feeling. It's sometimes a little anxiety-making because I think I could do something with my life but also by the same process, or paradoxical process really, work has come to me because I've given up trying. I've given up the intensity, and that's only over the last eighteen months really, and I have a lot of fun in what I do now.' It seems to come easy to me. The actual process of acting is very easy for me now and my motto has become, 'No sweat, no big deal and expect nothing.' And for me at the moment it works. I was never interested in the Everests. You know they all talk grandly about the Everest of *King Lear* or the Everest of *Hamlet* and all that stuff which is fine. I'm sure there's a truism there that to tackle those big parts you need to conquer a vast mountain of some kind. But I've realised now that I never really belonged in that world. I always felt alien in the world of acting because I couldn't actually convince myself that it was important and I thought well there's something wrong, I must make myself feel that this is important, I must make myself do these parts, I must actually grasp hold of these things and do them because if I don't it means I'm not actually taking my life seriously. And since I've opened my hand and let go of it I suddenly realised that it was something I wasn't interested in anyway and that my life as an actor has been really a form of therapy because I sense, looking back, that it's been a opening of some Houdini locks to allow me to free myself of some sort of unutterable burden which seems to have finally fallen away from me. It's the oddest experience but it's there.

CLARE: Why was it acting? Do you think acting was an accident?

HOPKINS: I don't think it was an accident as such. I was born in the same town as Richard Burton and Burton had made it very big as an actor. He was a big star and I was in my adolescent years then and I didn't know Burton. I met him once in New York. But of course he was a shining light in Wales. I was trundling round with all my inadequacies and inner pain and loneliness and I yearned desperately to be something. I yearned to get out from where I was, not to escape a town or a piece of geography, nothing like that but to escape some deep discontent in myself, actually some deep dislike of myself. I just simply wanted to be very very accomplished. Actually I wanted to be very famous and that burned in me for years and years and years. I remember once I met Richard Burton. I went to his house to ask for his autograph when I was about fifteen. It was a Saturday morning and I went into his house. He was home from Hollywood with his first wife Sybil. I knocked at the door and I said 'Is Richard Burton in? I'd like his autograph.' So she said 'Come in' and there was this mighty movie star standing there shaving with an electric razor which was all very impressive. He looked very American and I'd always had this longing to go to America. Anyway he signed his autograph and he asked me who I was, where I was. Anyway I left. They were on their way to an international Rugby match in Cardiff and as I was walking over the hill this Jaguar passed me and Sybil was in the back. She waved. She didn't know who I was but I waved back. And I remember walking down the incline in Port Talbot and I thought, 'God I've got to do something with my life, I've got to get out of this dilemma that I'm in, I've got to get out of this shadowland that I'm living in.' I felt I was living in the outer circle somehow of my own consciousness.

CLARE: You mentioned that the death of your father was some kind of watershed.

HOPKINS: Yes, he was a very powerful man, he was an extraordinary character, he was a workaholic. He was a baker and he worked very hard. He was a boy who left school when he was thirteen and his father before him was a very strong powerful man, physically powerful and emotionally powerful man. They both were very emotionally powerful, passionate. My father's passion sometimes gave way to panic and despair. He had a sort of Willie Loman complex about himself. He always believed that he would fail. But he was a remarkable man and I loved him very much. He drove himself very hard to survive and to accomplish something in his life and I think he was largely frustrated by his struggles in a way. We were very close, in fact sometimes too close. He was very proud of what I did as an actor and he was very thrilled by it all and I think somehow it unsettled him as well a little. I used to go down to Wales and if we met after a few days we'd have a fight you know, we'd have a row and he was so very forceful he could press my buttons and sometimes you couldn't resist it.

He knew my weak spots. He'd say 'Oh that play you did wasn't much good was it, you know, a bit of a washout.' I can understand now looking back what that was. I think it was maybe I was doing what he had always wanted to do. I don't know, maybe there was some regret and he couldn't control that.

CLARE: Was he jealous?

HOPKINS: I don't know if he was jealous, no I wouldn't say that but I think he was confused by his own son's gift or whatever because he was a very creative man. In the last years of his life he started painting and he wanted to write desperately and maybe, maybe there was a resentment, you know the resentment of age over youth or relative youth then. He was very ill in the last year and I was with him. He was dying of heart disease so he was a very depressed man and he was very frightened. But we were close together in the end and when he died I remember going to the hospital to see him. I'd never seen a dead person before and there he was lying there and this was in 1981 and as I stood at the end of the bed I thought 'Isn't this extraordinary, what an extraordinary process this is.' I remember the doctor saying, 'Your father's just died.' I remember the paint on the wall and I remember the notice 'No Smoking Please' and then the doctor said, 'Your father's died' and I didn't feel anything. I felt very remote and as I went in and stood at the foot of the bed and I watched him there, I thought 'Isn't this extraordinary this great drama of life. And I'm not so hot either because one day this is the way I'll go.' And I suddenly thought that it's all a game, all of it seems to be a game, the whole of life is a game, some peculiar playing out of something, beyond my understanding, like some drama. I thought he's acting dead now. This is some great force of life which is now playing dead, playing possum and he's played his game and he's off into some kind of other state maybe, who knows. But it was quite an eye-opener and some months later I felt very depressed and angry about something. I was back in California and I went to a friend of mine and I said 'I feel so angry and depressed,' and I was in real

real anger, like I'd never felt before and I wondered if it was anything to do with my not drinking for some years. Maybe it was a mourning, a mourning for the bottle maybe and this friend of mine said 'Why don't you write your father a letter?' I said 'Write him a letter? He's dead.' He said, 'Write him a letter.' I said, 'He's dead.' He said, 'Well write him a letter. Who knows, you never know.' So I did. I wrote him a letter and I said, 'I know we had our differences but I just want to say you know I miss you and I love you very much, I'm sorry we had our spats now and again, but we had a great time as well, wherever you are I hope you're at peace.' Now it sounds terribly icky and sentimental, but a few days later I had this tremendous inrush of energy. I was living in Los Angeles and had a very potent or palpable awareness that I just had to give up the struggle with myself because I was going to give up acting, I was going to give up this, I was going to take my toys away and not play, a sort of adolescent tantrum really. And it was in an afternoon in the house and this sunlight came through the window and it was a really powerful realisation that I'd better get on with my life and I think it was accepting and seeing for the first time the meaning of mortality, the meaning of the finite nature of life and that I'd better get on with it and make up my mind to enjoy it. And from then on, it was 1982, I've endeavoured to recreate myself, to reconstruct myself because I've got so bored with being a melancholic Welshman. My wife said unwittingly one day (she helped me with this), she said 'Well maybe you're always going to be a bit depressed, because you are Welsh and you are an actor and actors are different.' I said 'Well how, why?' She said 'Well you know, you put yourself through the emotional hoop.' And I said 'I don't, I never do.' She said 'Oh come on.' But whatever she said I thought, well I'm going to break the rule. And my life has been one of breaking the pattern for myself all along the line. That's how I've been able to escape from myself, by breaking the preconceptions of myself that I've had of myself, or maybe one or two of my friends have had of me. And when she said that I'm a melancholic, maybe I'm always going to be depressed, I thought well I'm going to break her perception of what I am and from then on I've been acting, I think it's William James's philosophy isn't it – act as if and you will become – and the oddest thing is that it has been working. I think I've got a handle on it over the last couple of years.

CLARE: Do you get a little melancholic?

HOPKINS: Oh, not any more.

CLARE: But you did.

HOPKINS: I get melancholic if I hear beautiful music but that's a sort of nostalgia. I no longer buy into the thing that if you're talented you have to be miserable, that simplistic notion that you've got to be somehow tortured, miserable, and I don't believe that. I believe the freer one is from all that mental dross and awfulness, the freer one is to create. Now whether one's work is better or not it doesn't matter because I don't want to revert to that misery again, because it's heavy baggage. And I've got a few friends I tell the same thing, and they say, 'Well how do you do it?' I say 'Well act as if you're happy; if you're depressed act as if.' They say 'What are you talking about?' I say 'Well I'm an actor so I can act, so I can act and pretend that I'm something else, and the oddest thing is that you begin to con yourself into becoming another person.'

CLARE: When you say you act it, even though you're not necessarily feeling it just at that moment and you act it, what do you notice about people's responses, do they change too?

HOPKINS: They do, they do. I find that they do respond. They respond because they seem to want to be with me, they seem to have fun around me, because I don't want ever to go back to that moroseness again and I don't like being with people who are morose.

CLARE: How gloomy would you have got in the past? Did you ever get to the stage where you felt you just couldn't go on?

HOPKINS: Well, yes, I think because I had such a lust for life some years ago, I nearly drank myself to death, because life was constantly disappointing. I think that's the problem with drinkers, the problem drinkers, alcoholics.

CLARE: Why did you drink? What was it doing for you?

HOPKINS: Because I was an alcoholic. Well drink, booze, is very attractive and it's terrific stuff if you can handle it. I'm married to a woman who has a glass of sherry every night and that's fine for her and millions upon millions of normal people can actually do it, I can't. I guess it's a sort of poison, I don't know what it is. I can't have one, because that is not enough for me, I've got to have more and more and more.

CLARE: And did it do something for you?

HOPKINS: Oh, yes the first hit was terrific, you know you get the first scotch or the first beer . . .

CLARE: Now what did it do?

HOPKINS: Well it changed my environment around me and made me feel at ease. It made me feel like Humphrey Bogart or John Wayne. It made me feel as if I belonged. You know I always felt out of sorts, ever since I was a little kid and I remember the first time I started drinking, that wonderful feeling when it hits the centre and you think, 'Ah!' I always remember seeing Sinatra on the stage in Las Vegas, I remember he had a scotch and as he drunk it he went 'Aahh!' and the whole audience went 'Aahh' with him and I, I'd given up drink by this time, but I remember thinking 'I know that feeling, I know that if you can have that drink, and say, 'Oh isn't this terrific' then fine. But I couldn't do that. I had to have more of that deep level of belonging. But of course what happened, and there's a sting in the tail, I became addicted to it and I couldn't stop. I had to have more and more and more, which is a common addiction, and it finally kills you. I couldn't get enough. There was not enough booze in the world to satisfy me or put me at peace.

CLARE: Have you any idea why you stopped?

HOPKINS: Because I was dying. Because I was going nuts.

CLARE: But some do, as you know. You must have seen a few yourself.

HOPKINS: Oh yes, I've seen it, I've been to a few funerals. I've seen so much insanity with drinking and drugs.

CLARE: It's a sort of cliché really, I hear in the artistic world and I hear journalists or some actors say, 'Well you know

Bloggs he gave up the booze but he was never quite the same since.' There is an equation in other words of drinking and creativity. Did you come across that, did you fear it yourself?

HOPKINS: Well the people who say that have got the problem themselves. It actually makes them feel well, it makes them feel better. They say 'Ah, yes he's lost the edge you see, Hopkins,' so that means they can go on drinking. But I smile now because it's none of my business what they do so I don't give a hoot.

CLARE: Did you fear it yourself? Did you see some connection between keeping going and drinking?

HOPKINS: Yes I drank because I thought it would give me the edge. I thought it would give me the passion and violence and all that was required of me, I mistakenly thought was required of me.

CLARE: And that without it you mightn't cope?

HOPKINS: And without it I'd lose it, that without it I'd be nothing. But now, you see, whether I've lost the edge or not is immaterial to me because at least I'm alive and well and kicking and I'm happy. Whether the quality of my work has deteriorated or improved I don't know. I certainly function better as a human being. I just get up in the morning instead of coming to and I go to sleep at night instead of passing out. I'd rather that and be a very dull actor. So it's immaterial to me whether I'm good or bad as an actor. I said once in some paper that all actors are damaged goods. I suppose there's some truth in that. I certainly felt I was damaged goods.

CLARE: I saw you quoted as saying something some years ago to the effect that you were genetically maladjusted.

HOPKINS: Genetically maladjusted. Yes, those were the put-downs. I put down myself before anyone could, you know, get the boot in first. It is a self-defeating game you know – hurt myself before they can then that sort of disarms them, whoever they are – it's not a very profitable game to play with oneself.

CLARE: Would your mother have argued with this trend in you? You describe growing up an only child getting this negative feedback from school and to some extent from your father, because of his own doubts about the future. But your mother had some hopes. Would she have tuned into the fact that you were getting this reinforcement of negative views about yourself? Would she have tuned into the fact that Tony Hopkins was beginning to believe that he really was odd?

HOPKINS: Oh, yes she constantly believed and she'd still tell me today, 'Why do you want to put yourself down? Why do you say those things about yourself?'

CLARE: She would?

HOPKINS: So from an early age she'd say 'No you're fine, you're all right you know,' and my father said it as well. I mean he was just a worried man because I wasn't very bright at school. I reacted to all that for some reason. But you know I can say with all confidence that no one is to blame. I'm not to blame. No one is to blame for any of that stuff. I'm an over-reactor. I suppose I over-react. What I've had to learn over almost two decades now is to not react, because you're a slave if you over-react. You're a slave to your actions so I gradually slowly trained myself to not react. It's taken a long time. It's not easy having a rage and a temper. Now, gradually, I try to count about ten before I blow or write it down or write a note and then throw it in the waste-paper bin.

CLARE: Has that changed your interest in or attitude to the critics? Would you, as you were growing up, would you have been very sensitive to what people said about what you were doing?

HOPKINS: Oh, yes, I hated the critics, I hated them.

CLARE: But you would have read them?

HOPKINS: You know actors say we don't read them! I hated the critics. You see in the theatre if you're working and you've done a play and you've worked hard they can devastate you, and destroy what confidence you've got in a performance. I did a play in the West End recently, *M. Butterfly*, and they tore it apart. Some of the critics were OK. I thought after about a week, I thought 'This is it. I'm not going to do this any more. This is stupid.' If they criticise a film it doesn't matter because it's over and done with. I have done some bad films but it never affects me because it's done, it's forgotten and not there. It's just a series of photographs. So they can say what they like. I don't actually, physically have to stand there, feeling like a lemon of inadequacy so that's why I enjoy filming so much because it can't touch you. I don't believe in this thing that we have to take our punishment, you know stand on the stage like good British gentlemen, stiff upper lips and take this crass, vicious, personal attack from these eunuchs as a lot of them are, because they can't create anything themselves and they're impotent a lot of them, I mean spiritually or emotionally impotent. Because if they aren't why are they just writing things in the papers? So whatever they say about a film it's over and done with, they can't touch you. But on stage it does get to you.

CLARE: Would you go back to the stage?

HOPKINS: If it was a really good play and it was worth doing and it wasn't too long a run, yes. I'd like to work in American theatre. I enjoy that, it's new, it's not precious. But criticism has put me off going back to the theatre. I have to read things very carefully before I make any decisions about that.

CLARE: Was it your drinking or what was it that, that broke up your first marriage?

HOPKINS: Oh, well that's an area that I really don't want to go into. That was just a rather unfortunate mismatch that's all.

CLARE: Do you see your daughter?

HOPKINS: Yes it was my first marriage. I was drinking and I wasn't very pleasant and I think we were both a little ill-matched together. But we have produced this rather lovely daughter, Abigail, and I saw her recently. She came back into my life about four or five years ago, so I had a quick crash course in growing up! I've had to practise actually letting go, as they say in America, letting go and letting her get on with her life. I don't interfere with anything in her life. I can point the way to her sometimes. She said to me once, she said, 'Do you mind if I experiment with drugs?' I said, 'You can do what you like but don't bring them in the house because if you do I'll kick you out in the street, because I don't want any police raiding this house.' I said 'But I can give you some fairly good reasons why it's not very smart to do that.' But I said, 'You do whatever you like.' I think she was testing me. She's in America now and having a good time and enjoying her life.

CLARE: When you said you had to practise letting go that's surprising because in a sense she was gone and had come back into your life?

HOPKINS: Yes, well my instinct was to think 'How can I make up for lost time? I'll actually be a good father. How can I actually mould this girl?' But then I thought 'It's none of my business.' She wants to be an actress and she's studying at the Actors Studio in New York but I just had to let go of my opinions and judgements and let her get on with it.

CLARE: Were you, looking back, a very difficult person to live with?

HOPKINS: I'd had my moments. I was very difficult yes. I'd been difficult to work with many times, very difficult, very complicated and very unreasonable. I've hurt a few people and I've shouted and hollered at people. I've made amends as much as I can with a few people that I know. My wife tells me I'm not as difficult to live with as I used to be. I seem to have gone into neutral. I feel relaxed at home and in my life.

CLARE: How important in all of that was AA?

HOPKINS: Oh, it was the turning point of my life. It did a 180 degree job. I got into that in 1975. I'm breaking all the rules actually talking about AA but however, you've asked me so I can tell you. It's an anonymous programme but it is the most amazing philosophy because it's taught me over the last fifteen years to let go of my life, that my life is in fact none of my business and that you are none of my business, my wife is none of my business. And it has taught me to release people, not to try to run the world, not to try to run my own life in fact. It's the oddest, I mean it sounds crazy, it's like living life back to front, but it's about surrender.

Now, it's not a religious organisation but it is basically a philosophy.

CLARE: Though it has a notion of a higher power of some kind?

HOPKINS: Yes and people can either take that as a committee of other minds and other knowledge and more experience and they can use that as a power greater than themselves, or they can talk about God. I don't know what that is. I know that something quite remarkable happened to me fifteen years ago when I actually realised that I was beaten, and that I was utterly powerless over my addiction.

CLARE: Where were you then?

HOPKINS: I was in Los Angeles.

CLARE: What happened?

HOPKINS: Well I was just killing myself slowly and my wife had gone back to England to leave me, to die I guess, or sort myself out.

CLARE: This is your present wife in fact. She had married you some years before?

HOPKINS: Yes, about three or four years before and I think she thought she'd had enough really and she just got out of the way for Christmas 75 and came back to England. She'd had enough. She never nagged me but she'd had it, she was exhausted. And I met my match in Arizona. I'd driven all the way down there and back in a sort of semi-blackout. I could have killed somebody, and it was a series of incidents that woke me up. I'd driven the car while blacked out. I mean I couldn't remember where I'd been and it was a moment of enlightenment. I thought I could have killed somebody and I haven't. It's a wonder I'm alive, and I phoned up AA.

CLARE: How did you come to do that? You just looked up the phone book?

HOPKINS: Yes I looked up the phone book.

CLARE: You'd heard of AA?

HOPKINS: Yes I'd met a woman in New York who was in a play with me and I was really drinking myself under the stage at the time. In fact it was pretty awful. Some of the actors, they'd be on stage and they weren't sure what was going to happen because I was four paces behind everyone else and I was playing the lead, which is not the best way to be. They were very tolerant but there were a couple of scary moments. And this woman who was in the play, her name is Mary and she is an alcoholic, and she's in AA, she never interfered with my drinking but I did ask for a bit of advice and she told me about the organisation. I didn't want to know any more. I thought 'Well I'll do it on my own.' And I did successfully for six weeks. At the end of six weeks I thought 'Well, what's the big deal, you know, I've stopped drinking so obviously I don't have a problem?' So I took that inevitable beer or tequila or whatever it was and that was it.

CLARE: Because the problem was the usual thing – you couldn't face the notion of being an alcoholic?

HOPKINS: I was denying it all. That's the problem with it, you know, you're, as they say, 'in denial' and that's what kills so many people. And of course if you're functioning as I was, I was functioning as an actor, I was making money, I was getting on quite well, so I was in danger of being completely blind. So many people do drink themselves into the grave because they are functioning, they are successful in business or they're successful in acting or the arts or whatever they're doing and they don't see that the world is falling apart around them. I was dangerously near that but fortunately I was so scared when I went out to Los Angeles, I was so frightened by what was going on in my head, by the emotional and the beginnings of physical pain I was in, aches and pains in my chest, and I was terrified of dying and I thought I'm going to have a heart attack. I was a hypochondriac as well, but it was the pain in my head that was killing me and the loneliness and the isolation.

CLARE: Your wife going back to England, had that been a shock?

HOPKINS: Yes, that woke me up, that really woke me up. I thought 'I'm losing everything I've cherished, I'm about to throw away a whole career.' I could feel that the writing was on the wall. I came to the most skidding halt in front of a wall and it was 'Your time is up Tony you know.' So I phoned up AA and I went in and talked to them. I was going to talk to them. I wasn't going to be talked to. So I had on my best jacket, intellectual arrogance and all that and I walked in and I knew it was over. The oddest thing happened because I'd actually made that phone call, because I'd actually asked another human being, another person for help or some advice. I'd never asked anyone for advice before or for a pointer or a way or a suggestion and because I asked for something I felt that for the first time I was becoming human. The most dramatic thing happened. I was picked up that night and taken to a meeting and I met an actor who I'd worked with a few months before and he turned round and he said 'Hello Tony,' he said 'We've been waiting for you.' He knew I was one as well, and it was over, it was over. I realised I was in a room full of people who had felt all their lives as I'd felt all my life, ever since I was a little kid standing on the corner of the street with a hole blown through my guts, lonely and isolated. I realised that my drinking was really a symptom of a severe kind of personality or personal disorder, emotional disorder and my relief was that I didn't have to analyse that, that I didn't have to go into endless psychoanalysis. The oddest thing happened. I've never had a need to drink or want, a desire to drink, I've thought about it a few times, but I've never had a craving for it.

CLARE: Did you have any withdrawal symptoms when you stopped?

HOPKINS: No. Not really. I thought I saw a few moths flying around but that's about all. I wasn't quite like Ray Milland but I had the jumps. I was a bit twitchy. If the phone rang I'd jump. But it was a wonderful time actually because I was so scared and I was so in awe of what was happening to me and what was going on inside my head. I started breathing again, I could smell things, I could see things, I could hear things. I had all kinds of strange insights which I've mostly forgotten now. It was almost like learning a whole new way of living. Every day is an adventure. I wake up in the morning and it's like waking up with a stereo in my head and cinemascope, full MGM panavision you know it's all there. I'm fascinated by the process of being alive. I'm fascinated by the actual mechanism of getting out in the day and moving about and doing things, and I walk everywhere and I have a great drive to enjoy my life. I remember coming back to London from Los Angeles and somebody said to me, when I was doing a film, they said 'Oh you've probably lost your nerve, you'll never go back on stage.' Within a month of that conversation with this actor who said 'You've probably lost your nerve, you'll never go back on stage' I had a play from the National Theatre, David Hare's *Pravda*. It's a wonderful play and I was asked to play this great character Lambert Le Roux, this monstrous journalist. And when I read it, I thought 'That's terrific' and I checked with them. I said 'You want me to play this?' I thought now is the chance for me to prove to myself that I haven't lost my nerve, and I got on stage, did it and it was a big success. And I thought 'Well that's it, I've not lost my nerve so what do I do now?' And I did Lear and Antony and I wouldn't say I enjoyed them totally but they were interesting experiences, they were academic experiences really. It proved to me that I had a brain which functioned and I could remember a lot of lines.

CLARE: It was different to acting pre-AA?

HOPKINS: Yes it was, yes, because all I wanted to do at the end of the night was go home, I didn't want to go into the bar. I just wanted to go home and have a rest.

CLARE: Some say that one becomes dependent on AA. It becomes a major source of support and consolation?

HOPKINS: It's the mafia really because you don't get out and live. It's not a big price to pay. You know if you get out and leave it you will one day surely either go mad or drink or die again.

CLARE: Yes, so you stay in touch with it?

HOPKINS: All the time. I go to about five meetings a week.

CLARE: Wherever you are?

HOPKINS: Yes, because it's the best thing, the best deal in town. It's the best thing I've ever done. It's scot free. I don't have to pay anything really. It's given me my life back in tons. So if I'm an addict of AA so be it but I'd rather be addicted to that than what I was addicted to before.

CLARE: And at these meetings would you always say something?

HOPKINS: No. I'd sometimes sit and have a coffee, have a laugh. I was in one today and the meeting was broken up by some poor fellow who was ranting and raving. But you have a laugh and it's a very interesting life. You meet a lot of people who are extraordinary people, an amazing bunch of people when you're meeting addicts and alcoholics. They're great people. They're full of life. They're very noisy people. They have tremendous zest for living. Of course people say 'Oh you've become an addict of AA' but that's because it reassures them they don't need it. But yes I need AA. I need it and I love going to it because it's no problem for me now. I've been restored to a degree of sanity I suppose, whatever that means.

CLARE: Do you ever worry that it's too good? Where's the melancholic?

HOPKINS: I've left all that Welsh melancholic. I believe I deserve it.

CLARE: During your time in the United States, given the Californian community with its heavy emphasis on and acceptance of psychiatry, had you ever, yourself, come across psychiatry or been exposed to it or had it suggested to you that you go and see somebody?

HOPKINS: No, I've never been to therapy. I'm very interested.

CLARE: When you played Doctor Dysart in *Equus* did you yourself take a look at psychiatry, given that he was a psychiatrist?

HOPKINS: I read quite a lot of Freud and Jung.

CLARE: At that time were you drinking?

HOPKINS: Oh, yes, yes, like a fish and I was very alive. I was half hallucinating most of the time because I was drinking tequila by the bus load. But I had some pretty good insights at the time. I remember being sort of on fire all the time on stage. I was probably terrible! I read a lot. I read quite a lot of Freud and Jung and, who was the fashionable psychiatrist then?

CLARE: Laing?

HOPKINS: Yes. R. D. Laing, I read tomes of Laing. He's dead isn't he? He died of the same thing that I was dying of.

CLARE: Did you ever meet him?

HOPKINS: No, I'd like to have met him.

CLARE: Or see him?

HOPKINS: No never saw him.

CLARE: No. I ask that because once or twice in your recent film you reminded me of him but I didn't know whether you'd drawn on him?

HOPKINS: Hannibal Lecter? No I never met him.

CLARE: But you'd read him?

HOPKINS: I'd read him. I went through a stage when I thought maybe I needed a guru. I don't think I want that anymore, I've gone through that.

CLARE: Was there ever one?

HOPKINS: There was a man in Los Angeles called Chuck. I can't give his last name away because he was an alcoholic and he was an extraordinary old man. He used to speak a lot. He was in California and he was the man who influenced a lot of people like myself. His sole philosophy was one of surrender. I heard him on my first meeting. In fact he was extraordinary and I was convinced there was a halo round him. He had this wonderful voice and this wonderful laugh, a great sense of humour and he would say things. He said, you know, my life is none of my goddamn business. And I thought that guy's mad, he's got brain damage, but over the years it's made sense.

CLARE: What do you understand it to mean? That your life is none of your goddamn business?

HOPKINS: I don't know the reasons why I'm here. I've given up planning and I've given up projecting into the future. I live in a state of non-expectation. I gave up expecting everything of people, expecting everything of life and life comes up with so many surprises. I have a creed I suppose you could call it, and it goes something like this. I say to myself, I don't say it I think it, in the morning when I get out of bed or when I'm going through the day, that it's none of my business what people say of me or think of me. I am what I am and I do what I do, because that's the way it is. And we're not going anywhere and there is no sweat, no big deal, there's nothing to win, nothing to prove. Of myself I'm absolutely nothing, of myself I can do nothing, and that's a state of surrender of giving it over to the very force of life itself. The proof of the pudding is that my life has been pretty good for the last couple of years.

CLARE: Did you see yourself as a destructive person?

HOPKINS: Yes, very. I think it was just untamed energy really. The drinking didn't help it at all. I used to also be very frightened of my own tempers and anger against people and my own intolerance, a very intolerant person. I suppose it sounds like I've been sort of learning lessons all the time, sort of doggedly learning my ABCs of life. But it hasn't been like that at all. It hasn't been a study. It's been something that's happened by some form of osmosis I suppose.

CLARE: You're not a conventionally religious person?

HOPKINS: No. But I do accept or acknowledge a mighty force which is much bigger than myself, that is the very force of life. So I do for the sake of argument and semantics call it God, and I pay homage to this power which is so colossal and beyond my understanding.

CLARE: Are you still a very independent, somewhat solitary person?

HOPKINS: Yes I think so. I like people, I like being with people. I love going to parties now. I didn't used to, and I love doing that. I like all that now. I spend time with people but when I've had my fill I go away and live on my own, and I love driving and I love walking, and I love my own company. And my wife fortunately is the same. We both love our own company. We spend time together and then we go our separate ways and do our own thing and I go off to America and work and she likes staying at home, so it's pretty good.

CLARE: How important is she to this process?

HOPKINS: Oh, a tremendous importance. She would deny this of course but she's been instrumental in many ways, in a very powerful way, in changing my life because she was a power of example, somebody who had such an inborn wisdom. She's very bright, very clever and a very wise person. She's sort of terminally moderate in everything you know, she has a kind of terminal common sense about life. She says all the things to me that I should have learned years ago which I've had to learn in the last ten, fifteen years, things like, you know, letting go, leave it, don't chase after that thing, let go of that resentment or whatever. She does all that sort of automatically. She's not a saint although I've said that I'd put her in a museum when she dies! But she's lovely, you know, she's very very helpful to me.

CLARE: The reason I asked that is that some might have misunderstood you when you said 'Life's not my business, my wife's life is not my business' and so on, that there's an air of almost detached impersonality about it all.

HOPKINS: Yes it is detached, it is detached. And yet we come together by talking and I'll ask her advice. I'll say 'What do you think of this?' She'll say 'Well do you really want to do that?' and I say 'Well what do you think?' She says 'I don't think you ought to' and I really trust her. She's a very fast reader. For example she'll read a script. I'll say 'What do you think?' She says no. I say 'Really?' She says 'No. Don't do it. You don't need to do it.' And she will say 'You've got to do this one,' and I'll read it and I'll see what it is that attracted her and it's usually the thing that I would like to do, so she has been of tremendous help in that way.

CLARE: Do roles that call on that turbulence, that dark side, do they attract you particularly? You've played one or two and there is the most recent role. Do you know why you're fascinated by them?

HOPKINS: I understand them for some reason. I don't understand the motives but I intuitively understood Lecter as soon as I picked up the script. I knew him. I knew him so well. I knew how he looked, I knew how he moved, I knew his voice, I knew everything about him, but I don't mean I knew what motivated him. I just knew how to play him, I knew how to get into the skin of him.

CLARE: So leaving aside what he did, you knew how he expressed his feelings?

HOPKINS: Yes.

CLARE: What's interesting about the way you do that role is that you suggest by complete control of emotion a very dangerous emotion. Is there something of that in you?

HOPKINS: Yes, I don't like displays of emotion. I don't like it because I am very passionate and I am very warm-hearted and I do hug people and all that. I've got that kind of propensity in myself.

CLARE: But you feel bad about the explosive displays of energy?

HOPKINS: Yes. I hate sentimentality. I loathe sentimentality, and cloying emotions. I have a reaction I think to what is inherently Welsh warmth, and the Welsh are very tactile people. They love touching and hugging and that's fine and I don't deny that, but it's something that slightly makes me feel suffocated.

CLARE: Did anybody ever do it to you? Was yours a particularly affectionate or physically affectionate family?

HOPKINS: Especially my mother's side yes. I don't like displays of grief, I'm ashamed of it, I'm ashamed. I have been ashamed of emotions. Emotions irritate me because they take over unexpectedly and I'd love to be in control of those and very often I'm not. I find them treacherous.

CLARE: And you're drawn to a character that appears to have that mastery.

HOPKINS: Oh, yes, I think what I've found tremendously attractive about Lecter is not that he's a killer, that was academic, that's just a part of his nature. What I admired about him was his absolute skill and penetration and his power of penetration, and his power of being the joker. Because that's what Lecter is, he's a joker. That was what Lambert Le Roux was really. There's a peculiar freedom in those characters because they have no morality, they are Machiavellian, they have no scruples about anything. The audience seemed to respond to ideas and things that Lambert Le Roux spoke which are very unfashionable, terribly unfashionable the things he says, as Lecter indeed says things that are very unfashionable. Lecter says diabolical things but the audience seemed to be drawn into it. I suspect in my layman's way that it's because we yearn to be free like that, to express ourselves that way. We had a prime minister who was like that. I think that's why people were horrified and at the same time mesmerised because she didn't care who was looking over her shoulder at her copy book, she didn't care, and that's what made her mesmeric and repellent. I think that's why every so often a nation responds to somebody who has no doubts.

CLARE: Now, this comes from a man who, up to what Americans would call transformation, this change, would have cared a great deal about all sorts of things. You would have cared what people thought, what they felt, what they said about you. You were far from being free in that sense. Lecter doesn't care. He is his own master.

HOPKINS: He is his own master, and he's free, although he's locked up in prison.

CLARE: Lecter uses power when it's given to him in an extraordinarily violent way. Does that appeal to you? Do you influence or exercise power over other people?

HOPKINS: No I don't. I don't consciously and I don't want to. I used to want to. I was very interested in frightening people and being this and being that. It's extraordinary what happens, how much power actors have, you know, on screen or stage but also in the simple environment of working on a film set and it's very interesting to watch how actors do abuse that power. Of course directors abuse power mercilessly but some don't, and some are very good directors and there are some good actors who don't exploit that tension. They will muscle down and get on with their work and make everyone feel comfortable. It sounds like I'm trying to be a very good man but I feel that's what I like to do – to make people feel at ease and not use and abuse power like I used to.

CLARE: One power of course is the power over an audience, which is part of the theatre, do you miss that? Did you enjoy it when you had it?

HOPKINS: I enjoyed it when I was good. I enjoyed it when they liked me. I didn't enjoy it when they didn't. I didn't enjoy it when I wasn't good in the part, if I was miscast.

CLARE: How important a motive is it for an actor, the response of an audience?

HOPKINS: Well it depends what you want to make of it. I mean some actors enjoy it, and I didn't. I used to take the audience as a challenge. The audience was a challenge to me and I found the theatre a big challenge and it made me very angry, or I responded angrily to the theatre, when I was on stage I was angry all the time. I remember in *Antony and Cleopatra*, I think poor Judi Dench didn't know what was going to happen next because I was very angry all the time. I found myself very angry and I couldn't understand what it was, whether it was the part of Antony which maybe, it could have been that there was a man who was thrashing around at the end of his life, everything was falling to pieces around him, he was a very angry man but I couldn't actually divide my own violent anger that kept coming up from my own peculiar past whatever that was, all those, those shadows kept coming back from the past.

CLARE: This is in your dry period, this is since you've given up alcohol?

HOPKINS: Oh yes, yes and it was that feeling of inadequacy, I'd go on stage at night and I'd stand there you know as Antony or Lear or whatever and I'd hear this little voice saying 'You think you're sexy in this part or you think you're good, you're pathetic.' And I thought 'I can't go on like this. I don't want to go through this anymore,' I thought. I'm not a masochist anymore. I think I was. I think I enjoyed all the pain and suffering of it all you know and it was a role I was playing, it was a role that a lot of actors play. It's a role I certainly played of being rather moody and introspective and misunderstood, and I was bored out of my skull with that role I'd played all of my life. And I was bored with all that past, which I'd only manufactured anyway. I didn't have a uniquely sort of depressing past. I'd a rather good upbringing. My parents were loving parents. I was treated well and they tried within their circumstances to give me a good education which I wasn't up to. So they did all they could for me. But it was just my own peculiar reaction to myself and when I was working in the theatre, especially in the classics, I always felt I was back in school. I'd never been able to throw that off. It may offend some people who worked with me and trusted me, but the fact was that I can't help that feeling, that was with me. Maybe I'll go one day. Maybe I'll venture back and do some work in the theatre.

CLARE: Yet the way you describe acting, it sounds that you draw heavily on your own personal emotional reservoir?

HOPKINS: Yes, yes all the time, I've been able to draw on some energy and some anger and some whatever it was, some very deep-seated and violent energy.

CLARE: Do you still do that? With Lecter, did you do that?

HOPKINS: Yes, but what I enjoyed about that was the actual control of it and actually being able to frighten somebody through a thick glass window. I was able to do that because I knew and I know what can frighten people and it was something that could frighten me. The first time Jodie Foster comes into the cell and sees me I'm standing there waiting for her, I say good morning, and I knew somehow that that would be frightening. The director had said 'How would you like to be discovered?' He said 'We've given you a big build-up, and now she's going to meet you.' I said 'I'd just like to be standing here waiting for her and she comes to the cell, that would make her jump out of her skin.' I don't know why but I know what scares. I knew that voice would scare people, because it scared me. I mean when I heard it I thought 'Oh, yes,' so I thought I can do that and I don't know what it was, it was something darkly romantic about it as well. There's a line that's kept haunting me 'I'll help you catch him Clarice,' and I had this vision of a man down the end of a dark long tunnel and she's in there with a little torchlight and this voice comes out of the dark ... It says 'I'll help you catch him Clarice,' like a sort of 'Speak your weight' voice and I find that disembodiedness so thrilling and strangely romantic. So I think that's what he was, he was a romantic dark angel to her, her guide, and a destructive fiend.

CLARE: Do you relate differently to women?

HOPKINS: Now? I like women very much yes, I do. Before I was rather contemptuous and frightened and angry at women and that's gone. Don't ask me how all these things have happened, but they have.

CLARE: You played a character in *A Chorus of Disapproval* and I wondered where that came from because it is so different from many of the others.

HOPKINS: That was sort of loosely based on my father, I mean my father, God rest his soul, my father was like that in a way. He wasn't as monstrous as Dafyd. He wasn't monstrous at all, but he was a very volcanic man. He had tremendous passions and he was a great storyteller, had a great sense of the dramatic. He should have been an actor or a writer. There was a lot of buttoned-up fury in him. One day, I didn't know how I was going to play the part, and I went up to Yorkshire to start the film. I went into the wardrobe department and they gave me these clothes to wear and these ties and I had no idea how to play him. I'd learned the part, I'd learned the text, learned the script, and I was in the wardrobe and I said, 'Well I don't know what I'm going to do.' I had a pair of old suede shoes on and I remember my father had suede shoes and he worked in a pub for a while, he owned a pub for a while, and they were always soaking in beer, when he was changing the barrels. And I looked down and I thought 'God they remind me of my father's.' And there was a coat hanging in the wardrobe, a short duffel, no a military coat and I put it on and there was one button missing and it was far too tight. They said 'It's a bit too tight.' I said 'That's it.' And as I started walking down the street I felt myself limping. My father had an arthritic knee and I thought 'I know this character, it's my father.' And that was on the first morning of filming and I was going down the street to knock at the landlady's house and I thought 'In for a penny, in for a pound, this is where I've got to play it this way.' You know when you've committed yourself to the film in this first scene that's it, you can't go back then. And I thought 'I've got it, I've got it,' and I had work glasses and I couldn't see out of one of the lenses because it was so spotted. 'This is my father,' I thought, 'Dick Hopkins has come home to roost at last.' And I felt he was sitting on my shoulder and I kept laughing. It was the first comedy I'd ever played. It was pretty ham-handed comedy that I did, but I enjoyed it, I had a whale of a time. Working with Michael Winner was pretty interesting as well because he's as ferocious as my father was, an extraordinary character, a bit of fun.

CLARE: It's a cannibalistic activity in many ways, acting. You chew up all these bits and pieces that are buried in your subconscious.

HOPKINS: Yes, well I don't know what it's about really. I mean, somebody asked me the other day 'How do you prepare?' I said 'I don't know, I just learn the lines and show up.' He said 'You must do something more than that.' And I said, Henry Wilcox, for example, I went for a make-up test when I was doing this part in *Howards End* and the make-up girl said to me 'Now we've got a moustache here to wear. You don't have to.' I said 'No, I don't think I want to.' She said 'Would you like to try it on?' I didn't know what I was going to do with this part so I stuck this moustache on and I said 'That's it, that's him,' so the moustache played the part. I didn't do any work I just learned the lines. It's an odd process. I suppose I'm a rather externalised actor, a mask actor. I have to know what I look like. I have to know what I walk like as the character. Beyond that I don't understand any of it which makes my life very easy as an actor. I try and keep it as light as possible, even old Hannibal Lecter. I remember the first day filming that prison scene when Jodie Foster meets me, and they'd been filming about four weeks before in other scenes. I thought 'This is it, you know, this strange limey actor coming over from England to play this part.' We started the rehearsal and my voice came out and they said 'OK let's shoot it.' So we shot the first scene. Jonathan Demme said 'Yes that's great, let's do one more take,' and I thought 'I wonder if this is working.' Then

Demme said to the guys working on the props, he said 'OK you can let him out now.' So they opened the glass door to the cage I was in and a man called Billy came in. He was an electrician and he came in and I said 'What are you doing in my cell Billy?' using my Lecter voice, and he backed out of the cell and I thought 'It works!' and so I knew I'd got the key of the character. It's all a bag of tricks really, there's nothing special about acting. There's no mystery unless you want to make it a mystery but it's a bag of tricks.

CLARE: Can you let a character go?

HOPKINS: It's never with me. It's a switch on, switch off, like a water tap. I mean Lecter – that was so easy because once the camera switched off I was Tony Hopkins again. But say 'Action' and Hannibal Lecter would come back. It's all very conscious. It's not a first form of schizophrenia!

CLARE: And you didn't have to enter into the mind of this killer or work out why he indulged these kind of impulses? Some actors do that kind of thing. They study serial killers. They go and meet a few.

HOPKINS: I find that very arduous and laborious. I'm sure they get a great deal from it, actors like Robert DeNiro, people like that, they're wonderful actors. I find that rather arduous. I'm either gifted or blessed with a gift for mimicry because I've always been a mimic ever since I was a child. I can keep myself open physically and mentally . . . and close my eyes and I get glimpses of this strange little ghost, whoever this character is and I get a vague sketch of him in my mind and I listen for him. So I can hear him speak as I heard with Lecter and all I've got to do then is fit an impersonation into this inner vision or this inner image of the man which doesn't take at all any effort really. It can take a few seconds or maybe take about half an hour of sorting it out. Once you've got it, you've got it. I remember with *Pravda* the same process of seeing the man very quickly. I saw him surrounded by darkness as if he had come out of the dark lagoon of everyone's nightmares, this monstrous man, and I saw him surrounded in darkness, this huge ogre, this dinosaur and I saw him clanking around in my dreams a bit and

I thought well that's what I'll do, I'll make him a monster. I'll make him some kind of terrifying charismatic dinosaur and what the actor, what I do is try and fit myself into it. Sometimes it doesn't work. I have great problems with Lear and *Antony and Cleopatra*. I couldn't find the mask, the look of the person, so it made it a rather painful process because I didn't know what I was doing most of the time.

CLARE: You couldn't find an Antony?

HOPKINS: I couldn't really, no. I found the drunk in him, I found the degenerate and confused baffled man who'd come through with glory and was at the end of his great career, and I could understand that.

CLARE: What could you not find?

HOPKINS: I couldn't actually find the core of the man. I've been told it is a very difficult part, a lot of people have come a cropper in it. Lear is also a very difficult part. Some actors have succeeded and many have failed. I sort of started off as a failure in it but gradually put it together myself as the production went on. I thought 'I've got to find a way of doing it,' but I started off on the wrong foot. I think I'd wrong-footed myself, I don't know how.

CLARE: Given your philosophy that you know your life is not your own business, do you take it as it comes or do you have plans? Do you make plans? Do you say there are things that you want to do before you die, for example?

HOPKINS: No, there's nothing I want to do. If somebody asked me what you want to do next in the theatre I say I've no idea so I take what comes. I remember I was doing *M. Butterfly* in the theatre and one afternoon I thought 'I'd love to do a nice movie or something. It'll be nice to go to America and do a movie.' I thought 'Well that's probably never going to happen.' I got into the theatre that afternoon. My agent phoned me. She said 'I've got a wonderful movie for you to do when you've finished the play. *The Silence of the Lambs.*' It came from out of nowhere.

CLARE: Do you believe in fate?

HOPKINS: Yes, fate. I don't know if we are responsible for the reality around us. We envisage something happening or we vision something in our lives or see an image of something we want or desire and it has an uncanny way of coming to us and it can be positive or negative. It's like a person says 'Oh it's bound to rain today' and sure enough it'll rain on them. I've learned to say 'Well it's not going to rain, I'm going to do something else with my life.'

CLARE: So this process of detachment, would it affect all sorts of things? For example there will be much talk over the next few months about next year's Oscars. Is that something that would interest you, that you'd care much about?

HOPKINS: Of course it would be lovely to be nominated, but even lovelier to get one. You know people say, and the Americans especially say, 'Tony, next year you're going to get the Oscar.' I say 'Oh yes.' The Americans love projecting and thinking about things and controlling the future. That's what's so exciting about working there sometimes. I say 'Well we'll see.' Of course I'd love to be nominated, and I'd love to get one, I'd be deeply dishonest if I said I wouldn't. Of course I love all that, I love all the glitz and the glamour of it and I love all the publicity, it's a great deal of fun. The extraordinary thing is I feel paradoxically slightly sort of disappointed because I'd always wanted to do a successful film like *The Silence of the Lambs*, to be in a sort of box office hit. I'd always wanted that. Ten years ago if it had happened I don't know what would have happened, but I'd had some vague idea of how it would affect my life and what I would behave like. Now that this film has come along and is a tremendous hit it's all rather anti-climactic. I'm thrilled with it, I'm pleased but I'm detached. I feel like a one-dimensional man. It's like nothing to do with me anymore. I wish I could feel excited and jump up and down. The oddest things have happened. I start reading the trade figures of the box office. I haven't got a cut of it or anything but I keep reading it and think 'Oh my goodness, it has made 122 million dollars there' and I don't know why I'm pleased because I'm not getting a penny of that. But I think 'Isn't that wonderful, I'm in a 122 million dollar film,' and it's fun, it's a lot of fun that. I went with a friend of mine called Terry and we went and drove in the car to Leicester Square two nights after it had opened. I looked up and I thought 'There it is.' And he said 'What do you feel about it?' I said 'I don't know, it's very odd – Jodie Foster, Anthony Hopkins – it doesn't make any sense any of it.' And I just smile, it makes me laugh, it makes me feel free.

CLARE: What's happened to the fear? Take the hypochondriasis you mentioned. You used to be very worried about your health and aches and pains, what's happened to that?

HOPKINS: That seems to have gone. You know I exercise a lot, I run and jog, try and take care of my diet.

CLARE: Are any fears left?

HOPKINS: I think the only anxiety I have is that all this may be an illusion and that this feeling that I have now may suddenly all vanish and I may revert to type as I was ten years ago, that I may become depressed. But no I don't have any fears. I have a horror of waste, I loathe wasting things like water and electricity and energy. I'm a bit of a miser. I can't bear seeing people wasting water and wasting paper. I can't bear to waste paper. The amount of paper we waste, and yet I've got a lot of books at home and that's a lot of wasted paper. I'm very generous with money, I love, you know, picking up the bill. I have been a perfectionist but I'm not any more, because that's the way, I think, to total madness. Perfectionism is when you try to live in perfect castles that you've built in the air, you know, and I used to do that. I used to be in rehearsals three hours before anyone else, when I used to work at the BBC doing *War and Peace* or at the National. Not the new National, this is going back some years, I used to be in rehearsals at seven o'clock in the morning, while the cleaners were going round so I could actually learn my script and actually work it all out before they got into rehearsal at ten o'clock, so that's three hours, all in order that nobody could pull one over on me. Now that's not very healthy, so I've given that up. But I've got perfectionist quirks in me. I'm on the jogging machine or I go running and expect to see reflected in the window in front of me a twenty-three-year-old young man, which is a bit silly but . . .

CLARE: Do you think much about your own death?

HOPKINS: No. I accept it. Carl Jung says there comes a point in our life when we have to stare our mortality in the face directly and come to terms with it and find either a faith or a good marriage or a job or work that you enjoy. It's very comforting actually because I do see that now. If this is it, if there's nothing beyond death and nobody ever knows that question then we'd better enjoy it now, and maybe, who knows, maybe there is something beyond, maybe there is something afterwards, no one can prove it and if that is so then this is an illusion so you may as well enjoy it anyway, so we've got it both ways. I keep a mild faith and I have a lot of doubt. Sometimes I believe and sometimes I don't believe. But I think Tennyson said something like that the best faith is to have honest doubt, which is better than all the creeds. This is the big event. It's no longer the rehearsal as I used to think for years, it was the rehearsal and that one day the big event would happen, my life would then get into session. And somebody whispered to me once, 'Tony this is it, this is the big event, you're on, this, this is the show, today and you're throwing it down the drain,' or words to that effect and that startled me. Now I love every day, I enjoy my life so much, and I've got a few good friends in AA. They ask me for advice and I ask them for advice. One friend of mine says to me sometimes, he says 'I feel a bit down.' I say 'Well don't get down, get up, you know do this, do that.' And he says 'Yes but it's all very well.' I said 'No, well don't ask me then, get on with it.' We have the power within ourselves. It's strange to say that since we are powerless, but we do have that inner resource which is I suppose what Christ taught about the kingdom within. So we have the power for our own happiness, because finally we can't look to anyone else for our own happiness. Nobody else possesses the power to make us happy or unhappy. It's a wonderful truth really. I am the maker of my own happiness, I'm the maker of my own life, the maker of my own destiny, the maker of my own good fortune. It sounds a rather Thatcherite or kind of callous way of looking at life, but finally that's it. Get on with it. My creed is get on with it. But I have been very blessed anyway. I'm blessed I suppose to find a loophole, find an escape hatch from the addiction and destructive side of my life and to find an escape hatch through this complicated submarine I was riding in, and I've found a way out into the open air and I don't want ever ever to look back or to go back. If somebody phones me up and says 'I'm feeling depressed,' I say 'Why, are you homeless? Have you got leukaemia?' And if they say 'No,' I say 'Well, stop it.' They say 'My job is affecting me.' I say 'Don't let it affect you. Get out of the job or find something, just something positive in life.'

P. D. James

The women crime writers I have met – Ruth Rendell, Patricia Highsmith, P. D. James – are all cool, courteous, imperturbable women in contrast to the contents of their books which teem with passion, disinhibition, violence. P. D. James is herself rather intrigued by this paradox which was one of the reasons I wanted to interview her and from the outset it proved to be a discussion point of some significance. What is of interest is that whereas someone like Anthony Hopkins muses over who is he and finds himself playing a bewildering variety of roles in a struggle to find out, P. D. James has had from her earliest years a very secure sense of herself, seeing the world as basically a friendly place and believing that people on the whole are going to like and accept her. Borrowing from the theories and the terminologies of the previous chapter, the cognitions she has utilised in her life have all been strikingly positive. She is fundamentally optimistic. She expects that tomorrow is going to be better. It hasn't of course always been so yet, despite a tragedy such as the illness and death of her husband, her positive view of life remains unshaken.

So why did she develop a positive self-image when Anthony Hopkins from a not dissimilar background could only feel self-disgust? She would point to the importance of genes. There is too the fact that how girls and boys respond to a critical or unsympathetic father and a supportive and affectionate mother differ. Her mother clearly influenced her, helped her, protected her perhaps from the full impact of her father's character and personality in a way that would have been more difficult had she been a boy. P. D. James does not equivocate in her description of her early childhood – it was, she says, a time of almost constant anxiety. Her dreams strongly suggest her main method of coping – strong defences, an emphasis on control. She refers to Anthony Storr's view that creativity represents

the successful resolution of internal conflicts[1] although in
fairness to Storr he remained doubtful that the Freudian
interpretation of creativity – as essentially the sublimation of
the most primitive infantile enjoyments and the simultaneous
denial of them – was true. Storr, I feel sure, would share
James's view that the writer does not need to 'have as much
trauma in early life as he or she can bear without breaking'.
The fact remains that she feels the experiences of her early
childhood were important for her.

But trying to identify this or that influence as the cause of
this or that trait, much beloved of classical analysis, is not
unlike trying to decide who committed the crime in a detective
thriller. In 1984, my former teacher at the Institute of Psychiatry, Professor Michael Shepherd, delivered a lecture pro-
vocatively entitled 'Sherlock Holmes and the Case of Dr Freud'[2]
in which he argued that the link between the fictional detective
and the real-life psychoanalyst is that both embody myths, the
myth of deduction of major conclusions from the identification
and interpretation of minutiae, the myth of scientific objectivity
and the myth of professional omnipotence. P. D. James's
detective, working with a little objective evidence and
resourceful brain, tames the outrageous breach of nature that
is crime and restores society to order and stability. The Freudian
psychoanalyst does much the same. Both are engaged on a
mission to unravel complexity, to contain irrationality.

Steven Marcus, in an exploration of the culture of psychoanalysis[3] has commented in detail on what Shepherd terms
'the Platonic bond' between Sherlock Holmes and Sigmund
Freud. 'A few years before Freud began his great work,' he
writes, 'another physician-writer made his appearance in
London. The work that he began to describe as being conducted
at 221B Baker Street makes for an interesting anticipation of

[1] *The Dynamics of Creation*, Anthony Storr, Secker & Warburg, London
1972.
[2] *Sherlock Holmes and the Case of Dr Freud*, Michael Shepherd, Tavistock
Publications, London 1985
[3] *Freud and The Culture of Psychoanalysis*, Steven Marcus, George Allen
& Unwin, London 1984

the activities that would shortly begin at the Berggasse.' Holmes's deductive method, his analysis of the most tenuous clues and connections, his scientific pretensions echo those of the founder of psychoanalysis. Another critic, Arnold Hauser, hammers home the similarities.[1] 'Psychoanalysis tries to detect stylistic character from accessories, from unobvious yet revealing details rather than from essentials. Being a kind of psychology of exposure, it follows up clues rather than plain and direct forms of expression and expects the artist to give himself away, more or less as a neurotic patient does.' The persistence of this mythical detective-psychiatrist is reflected in the regularity with which psychiatrists such as myself are often asked in social gatherings what judgements we are making of various persons from the style of their clothes, the range of their mannerisms or the tone of their speech! The notion of the psychiatrist as a kind of Sherlock Holmes or Adam Dalgliesh dies hard.

Making sense of an individual history can never be conclusive, is of its essence a matter of plausibility, of what appears to make sense. For example it seems likely that P. D. James's fear of destructiveness and violence owes something to the tensions between her parents but we cannot be sure. Indeed we would be wise not to make too much of any such connection given her insistence that her adolescence was relatively trouble-free and the fact that she appears to be free of unequivocal symptoms of panic or phobias. It has to be remembered too that many creative individuals quite welcome the suggestion that their childhoods were idiosyncratic or eccentric or in some way neurotic – it could even be said that while mental illness is generally the most unfashionable of illnesses, for the truly creative it could become an occupational necessity!

In P. D. James's case, the experience of mental illness has been second hand by way of her husband. A fan of her work, I had noted that on a number of occasions she had described dead bodies with a remarkable degree of vigour and detail. I

[1] *The Philosophy of Art History*, A. Hauser, Routledge & Kegan Paul, London, 1959

did not know until we met that she had found her own husband dead – hence my somewhat circuitous exploration of whether she drew on such a dreadful personal tragedy in her work. It might seem distasteful to some even to suggest such a thing yet I am continually astonished by the relentless creative way that some creative people do cannibalise virtually every and any experience for the sake of their art. In this case P. D. James didn't but given her sense of detachment, her ability to stand outside her emotions and observe like a detached, watchful surgeon, her acknowledgement of the 'splinter of ice' in many a writer's heart, I felt it legitimate to ask.

She quotes W. H. Auden on the moral probity of the classic detective story.[1] The fantasy which the detective story addict indulges in, Auden claimed, 'is the fantasy of being restored to the garden of Eden, to a state of innocence, where he may know love as love and not as the law. The driving force behind this daydream is a feeling of guilt, the cause of which is unknown to the dreamer. The fantasy of escape is the same, whether one explains the guilt in Christian, Freudian or any other terms.' Shepherd takes Auden's argument further and quoting Brigid Brophy in support reminds us that in a secularised era short of myths the detective story provides a new version of an old one, the central theme of which is a guilt which is rationally understood and whose cause is unravelled. 'On such foundations,' he suggests, 'Sherlock Holmes and Sigmund Freud – the archetypal detective and the protypical mental healer – are twinned as the contemporary heroes of an ancient legend.' They are indeed Nietzschean figures in their detached omniscience.

The fantasy which psychoanalysis underpins, so say some critics, is that it too promises a restoration to some Garden of Eden, to a state if not of perfection then certainly of completeness, of harmony where we may know love as love and not of law. Perhaps the individual sitting down in the psychiatrist's chair or lying on the analyst's couch can be compared with a

[1] *The Guilty Vicarage* in *The Dyer's Hand and Other Essays*, W. H. Auden, Faber & Faber, London 1963

crime to be solved, a case to be cracked. It is a tempting thought, a subversive one too but one surely to be resisted. In the case of psychotherapy, there are hardly ever enough clues and rarely is a cause identified with a certainty that would convince a court of law whatever about a detective story addict. But the excitement of the search is certainly common to the work of both detective and psychiatrist and there is too the promise of a moment of truth, an acknowledgement of the fact that yes, indeed, that was how it was, that is what happened, that is what made P. D. James what she is today. But unlike that moment when we put down the work of fiction, we can never be sure we have identified all the causes in the psychobiography, have tied up all the loose strings, have cracked the case even if, in pursuit and support of the myth, we sometimes appear to pretend we can.

CLARE: Phyllis Dorothy James was born in Oxford on August 3rd 1920. An Anglican upbringing in a childhood that was not particularly happy led to a job in an income tax office and a marriage at the age of twenty-one to a medical student. She has two daughters, Clare and Jane. Her husband came back from World War II with a mental illness, and after nearly twenty years as a psychiatric in-patient he died in 1964. By this time her career as a writer of detective thrillers had begun though in 1968 she subsequently became a civil servant. Her first book, *Cover her Face*, was published in 1962, and a steady stream of books has followed. She has won two Silver Daggers from the Crime Writer's Association for *Shroud for a Nightingale* and *The Black Tower*. *Shroud*, *Death of an Expert Witness* and *Devices and Desires* have been televised, while another book *An Unsuitable Job for a Woman* has been made into a film.

She is famous for creating two rather different characters, the professional detective, Adam Dalgliesh and the younger amateur, Cordelia Gray. In one of her books, Cordelia Gray wonders whether a preoccupation with human motives might not be one of the commonest human vanities. I asked her whether Cordelia Gray might be right?

JAMES: Oh, yes, I think she very well could be. It's certainly a great fascination to me, and I suppose there must be a fairly large element of vanity in it. Sometimes, I suspect that writers in particular stand as if they are rather apart from other human beings and observe them – watch them. This may be necessary. I'm not sure that it's altogether commendable sometimes.

CLARE: This sense of detachment is soemthing you've referred to on and off over the years. Is that something that's always been part of your character?

JAMES: Oh, very much so. From my earliest memories really. When I was a young child, my life was rather like a story. I would start telling it in the morning. I would say, 'Then she got up, and then she washed, and then it was time for her to go to school.' There seemed to be another person talking all the time about me. I felt in some of the worst moments of my life, some of the most traumatic, that I have been outside the experience, watching it, and sometimes I've wondered if there's any experience that could happen to me that I wouldn't be able to stand outside and look at. I then realised, of course, that would certainly be so if it were the death of one of my children, and also, I'm almost certain, if I myself were suffering great pain, which must be one of the things many of us fear, I'm sure I couldn't stand outside that.

CLARE: Is this standing outside ever an unpleasant experience?

JAMES: No. No I don't think it is on the whole. In a sense I suppose it's a rather reassuring one.

CLARE: Is it one that you can control, or does it just happen?

JAMES: I think I can control it to an extent, yes. Yes. But not altogether, not altogether.

CLARE: I'm rather intrigued. Psychiatrists often see people who describe something like that. The reason we see them is because they describe it as an unpleasant experience. It's even given a rather technical name – 'depersonalisation' – that is this ability to stand outside and watch yourself going through the motions. The reason that we see it as doctors is because the person complains of it. It's not something that the person can control.

JAMES: And I suppose they find it very frightening, because they can't control it, and therefore they begin to wonder whether they exist at all, or who they might be.

CLARE: Or why is it happening.

JAMES: Or why is it happening. No I think with me, as with many writers, it's totally different. Perhaps to that extent we can control it. I never feel as if I've lost, as it were, control of the situation. I feel I know who I am, and I know what I'm watching.

CLARE: But pressing it a little, the explanation that's advanced for this symptom is that it enables the individual to cope with things which otherwise would be very distressing, very overwhelming. So it happens, for instance, in anxiety-provoking situations. The person instead of becoming very anxious becomes quite detached. When you first noticed it, you say as a small child, was that a very anxious situation?

JAMES: Yes. I must say, I think of my childhood as being a time of considerable anxiety, but I'm wondering if that isn't true almost of any childhood. Sometimes people say, my dear mother used to say, it was the best time of her life. It was happy, it was wonderful. I find this very difficult to understand. It seems to me that childhood is full of trauma. I know for me, it was almost a constant anxiety.

CLARE: Why?

JAMES: Well, I think possibly because my parents were not very happily married. Looking back on the marriage now I can see with great sympathy what some of the problems must have been. It's so difficult in childhood, isn't it? You just cannot of course begin to appreciate perhaps the financial worries, problems of bringing up children, the overwork. My father was trapped in a job which he actively disliked. He was highly intelligent, but of course he was born at a time when that couldn't guarantee him very much of an education, or even the kind of job he would have liked, so he was a tax official and I know he hated it. He seemed to me a very cold man, and I think I was rather frightened of him.

Then in his later years, I grew very much to value the wonderful qualities he had, which were qualities of great courage, of intelligence, of humour, fortitude, independence. Of course when you're a young child I don't think those are the qualities in a parent which matter to you. I think you need other qualities. My mother, who was a very warm, loving, not very intelligent woman needed a great deal of demonstrative affection which she obviously didn't get. And this atmosphere, I think, did create for me a sense of unease, and I think of anxiety. I'm not sure that I was aware of it at the time. I can remember every night, I couldn't go to sleep unless I had imagined for myself an extraordinary kind of situation. We lived at Ludlow in Shropshire then and I imagined that there was this huge great building in the market square and lots of courtyards, each courtyard inside the other. There were beds in each courtyard. And in the innermost courtyard of all lots of beds and one of those was mine, and outside this fortress there were soldiers always all night walking down. And I'd lie in bed and think well this is where I am and once I'd imagined that then I could happily go to sleep.

CLARE: And if you couldn't?

JAMES: I always could imagine it.

CLARE: You mentioned that you were sometimes frightened of your father.

JAMES: Yes. I don't think physically frightened. I was frightened of his displeasure because I think my mother was very frightened of his displeasure, and I'm sure that we sensed this. I don't mean to make out that it was a desperately unhappy childhood, it wasn't, I tell myself, very often, that in a world in which, after all, three quarters of the human race, three quarters of the children or more, go physically hungry it was to that extent probably a privileged childhood. I didn't go hungry, and I had a roof over my head. But I certainly don't look back on it as being a happy time.

CLARE: You had two younger siblings. A brother and sister.

JAMES: Yes. We were nicely spaced. There were eighteen months between us. My father very much wanted a son. I was the first child. But I don't think I was particularly a disappointment because they'd been married three years – I was a very much wanted first child. And then my sister came eighteen months later when it was not very happy for her being both the middle child and the second girl. And then eighteen months after that came my brother, and that completed the family.

CLARE: Are their memories of those early years much the same as yours?

JAMES: Yes. I think they are. When we talk about it we can sort of laugh now, and conspire at some of it. The memories I think are very much the same.

CLARE: You mention somewhere that in a sense every writer has something of a trauma in childhood, or a traumatic childhood.

JAMES: Yes. I read somewhere, I can't remember where, that a writer should have as much trauma in early life as he or she can bear without breaking. I'm not sure that's necessarily true. But I believe it may have been true for me and that the writing has been therapeutic. It was a colleague of yours. Anthony Storr, who said that creativity was the successful resolution of internal conflicts. I suspect it is for me.

CLARE: You didn't start writing, though, till your forties.

JAMES: Very late. This is one of my regrets. It's a considerable regret. Then as I have this happy way of, as it were, either excusing myself or rationalising or justifying, I think well, perhaps I started when I was ready, and if I'd started earlier I might not have succeeded.

CLARE: The reason I say that is that I wonder what other ways you had of resolving your internal conflicts – if there's anything in that theory? Would you say for example that in your adolescence you placed a great deal of emphasis on order and security and control?

JAMES: Yes. Those things have always been very important to me. I think I'm deeply frightened of disorder and of violence. Certainly.

CLARE: Why? Why are you? I couldn't find much to suggest

that you'd actually had much personal contact with any of those things.

JAMES: No. No I haven't. I'm not sure why I am. I suppose I could say that freedom is tremendously important to me, and I don't think that there can be any freedom unless there is order. It was from an early age that I had this sense of order. I can't explain it actually. I can't say where it came from.

CLARE: You've written somewhere about your strong love of order. You said 'I suppose it may represent something of one's feeling that underneath all the order that is constructed by society, there's this great surging morass of violence. Of evil.' Can I just personalise that for a moment? Do you feel that underneath your personal sense of order and discipline that you have a personal violence or evil?

JAMES: I think I have a considerable amount of aggression. Yes. I don't know about violence. If I look back on my life I can't remember any act of violence against any human being, any animal.

CLARE: None?

JAMES: None, no, I can't. But I do recognise in myself the aggression. Yes. Yes it is there.

CLARE: How do you recognise it?

JAMES: Oh. I think in anger.

CLARE: Verbal?

JAMES: Verbal.

CLARE: Cutting?

JAMES: Quite cutting occasionally. Not often said to people who are going to be hurt by it, but expressed, spoken. Yes, there is a certain aggression there. I'm not sure when you say is there also evil. I think in theological terms there must be. The potential for evil is surely present in every single human being.

CLARE: Well, you say that. But that remains a theoretical statement about you unless you could point somewhere to where you might have teetered on the brink. I don't necessarily expect you to say 'Yes I can remember it' in this interview, but nonetheless, I suppose if I am pressing it that's what I would want to hear you say. You've been in touch with violence and evil in your writing. Some of your fictional creations exude evil and malevolence, or certainly destructiveness and violence. Do you ever feel like doing what your characters do?

JAMES: I am never tempted to do what my characters do. I do see murder as the unique crime. It is one for which one can never make reparation. I can't imagine myself planning deliberately to kill another human being. I can imagine myself killing another human being in self-defence, in defence of my children, or grandchildren. I think I have a healthy sense of self-preservation, but the deliberate planning, no. No I can't and I don't think there are very many people who can.

CLARE: Does violence disturb you?

JAMES: Very much.

CLARE: In what way?

JAMES: I suppose it wouldn't disturb me as much as it does disturb me if I weren't aware that there must be the seed of it in myself. I suppose because violence is so akin to cruelty. Cruelty seems to me almost the ultimate sin of one human being against another. It's very frightening. It's very terrifying, and violence does affect an order, and maybe one has a sense that civilisation and society is so extraordinarily fragile, that what we do with our legal system and our social systems and our policing, and indeed with every other aspect of our social lives is just to build very fragile bridges against an abyss of violence and disorder.

CLARE: I'm still thinking of that image that you mentioned right at the beginning of this interview – how you used to imagine, to get yourself to sleep, courtyards among courtyards leading to the central courtyard, a lot of beds, a community, a secure community with its guards. That is a very early image of anxiety and security, of order and potential chaos. You've very quickly tied a connection between how you are now and one of your earliest childhood memories, which makes me think that there's something about that early few years that really does hold the key to understanding a lot about what you've written and your coming to terms with things like murder and death. Let's look at your father. You describe him as fearful but not violent, so it was something else that frightened you. There's a coldness or a detachment about him I sense.

JAMES: Yes. I think there was. I was always very fond of him. I think I was probably his favourite child, except of course he very much valued his son, but I suspect I was his favourite child, as my sister was my mother's. And in later years, I was certainly very, very close to him. I felt that I understood him. But, certainly in early childhood, he didn't represent security to me. He represented anxiety but how much this was the effect of my mother's attitude to him I don't know.

CLARE: What was your mother's attitude to him?

JAMES: Oh. She obviously needed far more physical affection from him than she ever got, and I think she was slightly afraid of him, afraid of his displeasure.

CLARE: What was it like, his displeasure?

JAMES: I suppose it was really rather like a frost on the household, but we didn't actually see a tremendous lot of him. He was a keen golfer. He disappeared a lot, and then later, this was an odd thing, he didn't have his meals with us very much. He came home from the office and he would have his tray in the dining room and we would have our meals, when we were home from school, in the kitchen, so we didn't often eat together. So in one sense it wasn't that he was there so very much. I'm over-emphasising this. Maybe this wasn't at the core of these early anxieties. As I say I have tended to feel that they're common almost to every human being.

CLARE: But nonetheless, not every human being, certainly not in my experience, describes that powerful method of really self-relaxation that you had – the image of how you got yourself to sleep at night. Clearly not every child comes out of that environment and writes a whole string of successful detective stories either – though there's more to it than just the environment, don't misunderstand me. But one other thing you mentioned is your father's disappointment. That can often produce anxiety in a child as well – the fact that the father, or the mother for that matter, is not happy. I sensed in some of your descriptions that he was not a happy man.

JAMES: No. I don't think he was. As I say, he was a highly intelligent man. He was a musical man. He was forced to do a job which he obviously disliked. He did it, I think, very conscientiously, he was an incredibly conscientious man. However he didn't get promotion, and I suspect that was because he was a difficult man and he hadn't an easy personality. He probably didn't get the promotion that he deserved, and looking back on it, I've no doubt that he had to watch less able men becoming seniors over him. And, of course, he was in the First World War. He was very young and he was a machine gunner and he had a bad war. He ended up as a second lieutenant. I'm sure that did affect him very deeply so that I look back now on my father with great respect and great compassion and indeed on my mother too. It's so easy to judge when one is young. I think what a child wants is security and love, demonstrative love, and approval. I try to give my own daughters security, though that wasn't easy because of their father's illness, but love, and certainly approval, which I think we didn't always have. But looking back I'm sure they, my parents, had a far more difficult time, a far heavier load to bear than any child can understand and probably a heavier one than I understood until I was myself comparatively old.

CLARE: When did your father die?

JAMES: About six years ago.

CLARE: Did you have a relationship in latter years that would allow you to reflect with him on earlier years?

JAMES: No. We didn't. We didn't speak about childhood very much. And, I suppose this is strange, we never discussed things on this level. I suppose it's interesting that we didn't really. I was pausing there, because I was trying – merely wondering what we did discuss when I saw him. Family, and children and grandchildren. He was very fond of his grandchildren and very good with them, but rather superficially.

But we seldom talked about the past, except for the First World War. The older he got, the more he liked talking about that.

CLARE: And your mother – when did she die?

JAMES: She died about two years after my husband, and he died in 1964, so about 1966. She had a very unhappy old age, and a very cruel one. She had all sorts of disabilities, physical and mental, and she would have loved old age. She would have loved her grandchildren. She had a great capacity for being happy and I do feel a sense of resentment, which is a silly word to use, because against whom am I feeling this resentment, but as she had tried all her life to live what she saw as a good life, she was a very religious woman, she was denied those last years. However the last years of my parents were much happier than the early years had been, and I think this often happens in a marriage. That is probably one of the arguments for people persevering with marriages which they may otherwise feel are less than satisfactory. I think they could have had a very happy old age together, or a much happier old age together than ever would have seemed possible if she hadn't been ill. He did attempt to nurse her with considerable – well devotion is hardly the word – conscientious duty. Conscientious duty really, I think defined his life.

CLARE: Have you drawn on him. There's nothing of him in Dalgliesh?

JAMES: Nothing, not that I'm aware of, nothing at all. No.

CLARE: Not the detachment?

JAMES: I think the detachment in Dalgliesh is my detachment probably.

CLARE: You've led me to wonder which of the two of your parents you feel you resemble the more.

JAMES: I suspect my father. Yes, I think it has to be my father, though I think possibly the pleasanter side of my nature, assuming that there is one, no doubt comes from my mother. I value the attributes certainly that I've inherited from my father's side. I think the writing gift comes from outside. Any warmth that I have in my nature is from my mother and I didn't inherit my father's musical gifts, which were considerable. He had no opportunity to play. He wasn't taught – that wasn't the kind of childhood he had – but he had a very real appreciation of music. It was a great delight to him, and I certainly didn't inherit that. I mean, I love it, or I love some music, but I'm not musical.

CLARE: Were you an anxious adolescent?

JAMES: I don't think I was. Yes I was to an extent, it is silly to say I wasn't. It's just that I think of adolescence very much as being school days and I was very happy indeed at school.

CLARE: Could you have gone on to university?

JAMES: I would have loved to have gone on to university. This was before there was free university education. There really wasn't a chance of it, no.

CLARE: So you went straight into work?

JAMES: I went into work at sixteen. My brother went into the Air Force at sixteen, he was an apprentice, and then became a pilot when war broke out.

CLARE: When did you meet your husband? He was a medical student.

JAMES: Yes. I met him when he was at Cambridge. We lived at Cambridge.

CLARE: What sort of man was he?

JAMES: He was Anglo-Irish, an older man. He had very great charm which my younger daughter has inherited, though it's a very difficult thing to define, isn't it. It wasn't superficial. He had a sense of humour. He was intelligent in a rather eccentric way. He was eccentric. I'm not sure that he should have done medicine. In fact I'm sure he shouldn't.

CLARE: Why?

JAMES: I just don't think it was right for him. It was too much of a strain I think. In fact it's rather a silly thing to say but I have a feeling it wasn't right for him.

CLARE: He was still a student was he, when the war broke out?

JAMES: Yes he qualified fairly soon.

CLARE: He did.

JAMES: And I worked in the Food Office in Marylebone. He was at the Westminster Hospital and we lived in a very small flat in Marylebone Square, now bombed. Then I became pregnant and I went with my mother-in-law to a house in East Sheen.

CLARE: I was never clear quite how soon after he returned from the war that he became ill.

JAMES: He came back ill. He returned and it was fairly obvious he was behaving extremely oddly. It took a long time to diagnose but he never was mentally well from the time he came back, except for a few weeks at odd times with his father. He was in and out of psychiatric hospitals more than I care to name. No one really was able to help him. Life was difficult in that I seemed to be spending all my time giving long case histories to yet another psychiatrist. There was a feeling that they wanted to help him, but in the event no one did and he died in 1964, when he was forty-four.

CLARE: What happened?

JAMES: I found him dead.

CLARE: In hospital?

JAMES: No. No.

CLARE: At home?

JAMES: At home.

CLARE: And the detachment you mentioned, did it help you then?

JAMES: Yes. It did.

CLARE: You never drew on any of these experiences?

JAMES: No. No. Never.

CLARE: Not consciously anyway.

JAMES: Not consciously. I never wanted to. This may have been one of the reasons why my first book was a detective novel. I didn't want to write the usual autobiographical first novel, and I have never wanted to use my husband's illness or the more traumatic parts of my own life in fiction at all.

CLARE: Some writers are extremely autobiographical. They draw immensely on the well of their human experience.

JAMES: Yes. I was reading a book about C. P. Snow recently, a book in which he was answering questions by this journalist, and in effect identifying the characters, saying 'Yes, this character was so and so at Cambridge' and so on. Almost throughout *Strangers and Lovers* I think there wasn't a character in that sequence which he couldn't give the real life equivalent of. There seem to be two kinds of writers in this way, those who do use characters they've known in real life and I suppose their own experiences, and those who don't, or at least, who are not aware of doing so, or if they do, have the experience as it were somewhat filtered through the creative imagination. I'm certainly one of the second group.

CLARE: I'm a little thrown because one of the outstanding features of you as a writer is that you're not just obsessed with murder, but you're obsessed with death, and in a number of your books the discovery of a dead person is central. You've talked about it as central. You've talked about the removal of the dead body as changing a place. You've talked about the importance of that moment. And now you've told me that it happened to you.

JAMES: Comparatively late in my life. A lot of these books were written, or a number of them were certainly written before that event.

CLARE: It didn't change you, writing about it though.

JAMES: No, no.

CLARE: Did it affect you – writing about it?

JAMES: I don't think so.

CLARE: They're kept apart – the real experience and the fictional creation?

JAMES: Yes.

CLARE: Can they be?

JAMES: Well, I can only say it seems to me that they are.

CLARE: Yet, as a writer, when you're writing, you're attempting to create a truth.

JAMES: Yes, indeed, but I've never, ever used my own experience, never knowingly used, and I think it would have to be knowingly used, because you would have to be thinking back to that particular moment, whatever moment you were using in your real life, whether it were really a traumatic one, or a very terrifying one, you would have to be thinking back and saying 'That's what it looked like, that's what I felt like,' and I'm never aware of that. It's much more as if what

I'm describing already exists somewhere in a kind of limbo which must be, I suppose, in my imagination somewhere, and I'm getting in touch with it, and getting it down on paper in black and white. I'm not remembering what has happened to me. I'm getting in touch with what is happening to other people.

CLARE: You wondered whether detachment was a good or a bad thing.

JAMES: Well, I think someone said writers do have a splinter of ice in the heart, and I think that one does possibly. Perhaps I shouldn't speak for other writers, as if I'm suggesting that we are a rather heartless crew who observe and make use of other people's misfortunes. I don't think that is so, but certainly they have the ability to look at experience, one's own and to look at life. There is a certain amount of detachment and the danger is I think, and this is a danger with my character, Adam Dalgliesh, that one can make your work an excuse for non-involvement. He has one of his characters say that if you are a spectator it's a privileged position, but if you go on doing it long enough then you lose your soul. I think one should be involved in living as well as trying to distance oneself from experiencing, using one's own experience. Nevertheless, detachment does seem to me to be part of my writing equipment.

CLARE: In the years between the beginning of your husband's illness and his death you began your writing career. Your childen were reared. The impact of it all on you, do you think it exacerbated your sense of detachment, hypertrophied it? Do you think it made any difference to you? How did you cope with what was a fairly harrowing experience?

JAMES: I suppose I was able to cope for a number of reasons. One is, I think one's physical and psychological make-up for which one really can take no credit, nor indeed can one be blamed. I am basically optimistic. I basically pick myself up. I basically feel that tomorrow is going to be better. I basically feel at home in the world. I feel that despite early problems and difficulties for me the world is a friendly place. I feel that people on the whole are going to like and accept me, and help me. If they don't then I think this is where I have these feelings of revelation. I mean I am disproportionately upset by it. But on the whole this doesn't happen very often, so I have that optimism. I had two children. I loved them very dearly. I had the support of friends, of colleagues and of my parents-in-law. I feel on the whole probably I am a coper.

CLARE: Were you prepared for your husband's death?

JAMES: No. Not really.

CLARE: So it was a blow?

JAMES: Well, it was for him I suspect, and for me at the time, possibly a relief because he was not getting better. It has become a very long and increasing grief. It wasn't so much a blow at the time. Indeed it came at a time, a very difficult time and I'm not sure how much longer I could have coped really, because he was living then at home, and I was working full time and one would never quite know what one was coming home to. As you know there's an emphasis in psychiatry on so-called community care – releasing people from psychiatric hospitals into the community into a care which is usually not available for them, and it's something I feel very strongly about. I know that is another issue, but I'm simply saying that I don't think at the time it was grief. I was very upset, very upset, but what has interested me, is that I have continued to be upset. I have continued to grieve for him. I think that's because with the beginning of old age, I realised that now that I'm not short of money how much we could have done together, and how much he would have loved his grandchildren. Indeed, when he died there was the feeling that he had not seen his grandchildren. My first grandchild was born not so very long after. This was part of the grief at the time for him, and certainly I can still think of him now and find I am almost as distressed as I was in the weeks after he died. This has interested me.

CLARE: At times you describe your brain, your psyche as if it's compartmentalised, a bit like those courtyards. And yet when I listen to you speak I find it difficult to imagine how it works. First there is P. D. James writing about Dalgliesh, Cordelia Gray and various kinds of mayhem going on, and then there is your real life, which at times you say is much the same as everybody else's. Yet yours is emotionally a very colourful one. I mean it leaves much of what you've written academic in comparison.

JAMES: Oh yes, indeed it does. It does. Yes. I often feel it is my life in a sense that is in compartments. This seems to be represented in a way by my friends. I have friends who worked with me in the Health Service all those years ago. I have friends who worked with me at the Home Office. I have friends because they're writers. I have at least one friend who is a friend because she was at school with me. And they represent really different aspects of my life. Those who are not writers, some of them are not really interested in writing particularly, and I suppose they see a different side of me. Or perhaps in my relationship with them I am rather a different person than I am in my relationship with friends who are writers. It has seemed to me in the past that I have tended to live my life rather in these sorts of compartments. And then there is a compartment for being a mother and a grandmother, of course.

CLARE: Somebody, I think it was the actor who plays Dalgliesh, Roy Marsden, said of you that you were layers upon layers. Do you think you are particularly mystifying to others?

JAMES: I wonder. I think I must be mystifying to others because they look at me and say, as they say all over the world, how can a respectable middle-class English woman, especially a grandmother, write such terrible books about murder! This does seem to mystify them. I suppose this makes people feel that there must be a sinister depth somewhere, or a bottom layer perhaps, maybe one that's best not looked at too closely.

CLARE: Do you ever worry about being murdered?

JAMES: No. No. I think like any woman I can work myself into a state of anxiety if I'm alone, and if I look at the wrong thing on television late I can. But certainly as I get older this seems to worry me less. There's a feeling of, oh well, if it happens, it happens.

CLARE: Would you ever write some of your more chilling

material in situations like that, say being alone, late at night, at home.

JAMES: Oh yes. I could write it, because I'm never frightened of myself. It's reading what other people have written.

CLARE: Could you wander round a churchyard late at night?

JAMES: Yes. I'm not sure that I'd want to spend the night alone in a so-called haunted house.

CLARE: No. That is somewhat extreme.

JAMES: That is rather extreme isn't it. The thing is, it raises interesting questions because why shouldn't one? I mean, how many of us really believe in the existence of ghosts, so why don't we want to spend the night in a so-called haunted house? Apart from the discomfort, absence of lights . . .

CLARE: The reason I ask why you particularly is because of your imagination. I get the feeling that if you were put on a Dorset beach looking at a cliff you would immediately think of a poor disabled old man in a wheelchair being tossed over it. You have a very vivid imagination about violence. There are some people you could stick in a cemetery at twelve o'clock at night and they wouldn't have the imagination to think of anything other than a quick smoke. But you actually have a very vivid imagination of violence.

JAMES: Oh, yes. And in almost any situation. I must say the images that come into my mind tend to be images of death. I mean as an easy example, going round University College where they've got that box with the old philosopher in – Jeremy Bentham – and I believe he's opened up once a year; well when I was told this immediately I thought, 'Well, there you are, there's the beginning of a good book. He's opened up – but there isn't old mummified Jeremy in there at all, there's the unpopular senior lecturer, who could have a noose round his neck, or a dagger through his heart,' and I suppose this is the kind of way certainly in which my imagination does work, yes.

CLARE: I would have thought that as you wrote your material your own imagination would scare the living daylights out of you?

JAMES: Not at all, no. But you see this is where I think the detachment comes in. I was writing a chapter actually this morning, working on a chapter which is very, very chilling indeed. And I certainly felt it was chilling. I almost felt well I'm not sure if I hadn't written this I'd much like reading it. But I didn't frighten myself.

CLARE: And why did you write it?

JAMES: Well, it was a necessary part of the plot. I mean that is how it happened in this book. And that is how it seems. That is indeed how it happened. When, earlier, I was thinking of this chapter I had it happening quite another way, and then I realised that as I wrote it this morning so in fact it happened. This is getting back to the sense I have of a book, and the characters and the plot existing in their wholeness outside myself. The business of writing, the business of creation, is really getting in touch with them and getting them down on paper. So that you can sometimes even have the feeling, waking up in the morning, that of course it didn't happen like that. That conversation I've been working on took place the week earlier, and they were in quite a different place when that took place.

CLARE: Do you think that the genre in which you specialise is to bring people in touch with anxiety and threat who would otherwise pass it by? Do you think it is ultimately reassuring?

JAMES: Oh I think for most people it is ultimately reassuring. There may be many reasons why I write it but I suspect that I am attracted by the order of the genre, because it is very disciplined, it is very ordered, it is not self-indulgent, you know. It's structured, and I like that. As far as people reading the classical detective story, I feel that there are rather interesting psychological reasons why the genre continues to be popular. Although, you know, every decade the critics will prophesy the end. It was in 1890 in reviewing Sherlock Holmes the reviewer in Blackwoods magazine wrote that considering the difficulties of hitting on any fancy that is decently fresh surely this sensational business must shortly come to an end, and it goes on. And I feel that it is because it's a paradoxical genre. You do have violent death at the heart of your novel, and yet the novel discusses the fears, the terror, and enables people perhaps to come to terms with it although they may not realise that this is it. At one level I suppose it intellectualises death. It makes it into a puzzle.

CLARE: I wonder too whether in a strange way it makes death predictable and removes its arbitrariness? I notice that somewhere you were quoted as saying you know, that death by terrorists in the street, the sort of anonymous death is not the stuff of which this kind of genre is made, but it did strike me that that is much more the sort of death that any one of us will die, not necessarily being blown up in the street, but we'll die an abitrary death as a result of a disease, or an accident, or a mishap of some kind. Much death, indeed even the death that gets to the courts is obscure, is ambiguous, we never really know why Neilson killed all those people, we never really know why Sutcliffe did what he did.

JAMES: No there isn't an answer.

CLARE: There isn't an answer.

JAMES: And you see this is part of the attraction of the genre, that in one sense it dignifies death. It says that human life has a unique value and that this applies even to the least attractive, most disagreeable, most dangerous, most evil man. Everyone has a right to live his or her life to the last natural moment, but when murder takes place, the resources of the state, or the resources of this omnipotent great detective, the great private detective are brought to bear in order to bring the perpetrator to justice. It is a law and order affirming genre. At the same time you have a problem which at the end of the book is solved. So that in an age of anxiety, such as our own, when there are problems and social problems, racial problems, international problems, which despite all our goodwill and effort and resources and the money poured into them, do seem beyond our ability to solve, here at the end of these extraordinary books, the problem is solved. And it isn't solved by supernatural means. It is solved by human beings, by human intelligence, human relationships, human courage. What I think is interesting perhaps about my books, is that although the problem is solved, we don't have a restoration of order and goodness and normality. W. H.

Auden liked detective stories and he wrote in an essay called 'The Guilty Vicarage' that they should be set in a small town, or a village, because it had to be a great good place. It had to be an Eden and that murder had to be as disruptive as if the dog had made a mess on the drawing room carpet. And then at the end one has a restoration of order and peace and goodness again. I don't think in my books one does. I think in one Dalgliesh says 'It's a very contaminating crime,' that no one it touches remains unchanged, and very often at the end in fact, the people who have suffered most are not the guilty, but the innocent.

CLARE: What about the suggestion that it tames death?

JAMES: Oh, is it possible ever to tame death? I must say I think death is fascinating, because it's the one experience which we can't experience. I suppose you could argue that it doesn't exist for us really because we are not going to experience it are we, we are only going to experience dying, we are never going to be able to experience death.

CLARE: Can you remember your first acknowledgement of death's reality?

JAMES: Yes. I think it happened, how old would I be, probably nine, when I was paddling in Ludlow down by the weir and a child got drowned. I didn't see the child drown. We were all sort of hurried to one side and then sort of taken home and, weeks afterwards, one heard the adults whispering about the child. I think that was the first time when I realised that the child had been at school with me the day before and I had known her. I think I quite liked her. She wasn't a close friend, but she had seemed ordinary, unremarkable, and now she didn't exist anymore, and I was left wondering where she was, if she was anywhere. Of course as I'd had a conventionally religious Anglican upbringing I was expected to believe that she was in fact in heaven. I don't think it ever occurred to me that she was in heaven. I suspected she might be somewhere but it seemed to me to be a great mystery. But certainly then I began to get some idea of the absolute finality of it and that's difficult for a child to accept.

CLARE: You've mentioned your husband — were there any other personal contacts with death?

JAMES: No. I can't recall any. I can't think of anything in my own life, my early life, or subsequently that could possibly have lead to my interest in this kind of fiction. Although I would admit I'm interested in death, I think I'm even more fascinated by time. After all time and death are twins in a sense because death must be the end of our experience of time. Time intrigues me. Time is just so inexorable, so mysterious and so erratic and I've been interested in both, but I can't honestly point to any particular experience that could have lead to this.

CLARE: But you don't just write about murder and you don't just write about death, you describe the dead in an extrordinarily detailed way. I was struck by the fact that in I think it's in *An Unsuitable Job for a Woman* you describe Bernie Pride's death by suicide. In great detail, right down to the actual artery severed at the wrist, the blood-stain on the floor, how it was cleaned away, the body being discovered. I can't for the life of me remember why he did it, although there was an explanation of some sort, oblique, hinted at. Through the book you begin to piece together poor old Pride and his failure really to live up to that strange name. But the death was detailed. Reading it you might be tempted to say this woman's most morbid preoccupation is the dead!

JAMES: I'm attempting to write realistic books. I know that begs a lot of questions — how can they be realistic? — but then all fiction is artificial. I don't see that the detective story need be regarded as any more artificial than any other form of fiction. And assuming I am trying to write a fairly realistic book then it seems to me that the moment at which the body is discovered, whether in this case by the girl detective, or by one of the suspects or by one of the other characters in the book it's a tremendously important moment and I think I want the reader to see the horror and the shock through the eyes of the person discovering the body. It's a very important moment in the book, the moment that the body's discovered,

I think. One wants to be realistic about it. But I've never seen anyone who has died in that way.

CLARE: You haven't.

JAMES: Oh, no. If I need any details I do research. I use Keith Simpson's book on forensic medicine quite a lot to get the information. I just want it to be reasonably accurate. What's interesting to me I must say is that I can describe the bodies in my book, I hope as it were, realistically. But I could not write a scene of torture, nor in fact can I read them. Nor can I watch them on television or the screen. I've never been able to. They do upset me. But my victims are safely dead. Once they're safely dead they're not feeling. Then I seem to be able to stand outside and see what they look like. But to describe a human being deliberately inflicting pain on another, I couldn't do that. I find it very frightening, very terrifying.

CLARE: Do you think there is a beauty in the dead?

JAMES: No. I don't. I don't, and I wouldn't feel any attraction. I think there are people who just want to look at dead bodies or like looking at dead bodies. I can't see that at all. Once when I was in hospital administration I saw some dead bodies because I was concerned with taking exams on hospital building and planning and was doing some research on how one could plan a mortuary and I saw bodies there. One does have this feeling of the person having gone, of there being just a shell of just something outworn, outgrown, left behind. I don't think one has necessarily perhaps to be a religious person to feel that. No, I don't think they're particularly beautiful and I'm not, I think, sentimental. I find the Victorian obsession with death a bit repellent, the sentimentality of it, just as I'm out of sympathy with sort of euphemisms of sleeping, of rest. It all seems to me totally meaningless.

CLARE: Do you think much about your own death?

JAMES: Yes. I do, perhaps not as much as one should, at the age of nearly sixty-five. I think it's important to think about it occasionally, and to come to terms with the fact that it is going to happen. With luck there are so many years left but not all that number. I write very slowly you see. I write a book every three years. It's seldom quicker than that. If I end at seventy-five that is three more books. This is salutary. It's also important to remember it because I think it helps one to live one's life fully — and to look one's last on all things lovely.

CLARE: Do you look back on your life at this stage with regrets?

JAMES: Some regrets, but with far more gratitude. I think the basis of such religion as I have is gratitude. Gratitude for so much privilege, that I have known love, that I was born healthy, that I have a talent, that I have the energy to exercise it, that I have two daughters whom I love, grand-children whom I love, friends, no financial anxieties. This adds up to immense privilege, immense privilege. And I'm grateful for it.

CLARE: And the regrets?

JAMES: I wish I'd worked a little harder in youth. I wish I'd started writing earlier. To be over forty when one's first book is published, at my age it seems a waste of time. I wish I'd gone to university. I wish odd things. When the war broke out I wish I'd gone into one of the women's services. I didn't at the time because I was very much a pacifist and although I felt that war had to be fought, I thought I was better doing things like nursing which I was totally unsuited for.

CLARE: Why?

JAMES: Why am I unsuited for it?

CLARE: Yes.

JAMES: I'm not unsuited for it in a sort of domestic setting. I think I'm quite good at nursing people who are sick, but I'm certainly unsuited for it in the sort of institutional setting.

CLARE: An emotional failing?

JAMES: I just didn't enjoy it. I didn't like it. I think there are other things I could have done. I feel that there are experi-ences that would have been useful to me as a writer that I could have had if I'd a little more initiative. But it's not very sensible, I think, to look back and say here and there I have regrets because I'm never sure how much choice we do in fact have at the time when we make what seem to us later to have been choices.

CLARE: You mention religion quite a bit but I don't know how important it is to you. How does it help or not help in relation to this central preoccupation, this unease?

JAMES: I think I've probably come to terms with the unease. If I haven't I imagine I have and am fairly happy in that belief. I think it's important to me.

CLARE: Religious belief?

JAMES: Yes. I suspect religious belief is like an artistic sense. You have it or you haven't. It sometimes seems to me it doesn't have a great deal to do with conduct for example. It is a sense of a world other than this, and I think I would describe myself as basically religious, certainly a deist, a very imperfect Christian certainly.

CLARE: Do you believe in a hereafter? These dead bodies, are they somewhere else?

JAMES: I don't know. I was coming past the church here in Langham Place, and a sermon was advertised 'What will happen to you when you're dead?' it said. Someone is going to speak with some authority on it. It struck me as being very odd that someone, even a Christian priest, can think that he can speak with very much authority. I'm not sure that we should occupy our minds too much with the possibility of any existence after death.

CLARE: What are your anxieties?

JAMES: Not in fact, thank God, very many. I suppose I want an old age which is healthy so that I'm not a burden to my children or my grandchildren. I hope most of my life to be free of pain. Pain is something that I am very frightened of. Pain, a dreadful pain certainly, seems to be much worse than death, and in fact I'm sure that most human beings feel that. I would hope to be able eventually to die in dignity and in full possession of such faculties as I have. I have of course the wider anxieties which any human being must have now about the world and about the bomb. I'm less at home in my country than I used to be before the war of course. It's difficult to know really how much this is the nostalgic looking back of someone who is now becoming an old woman. I worry about some of the things I see happening. That's about it I think really.

CLARE: We started the interview talking about your detachment. At times through the interview there have been examples of that. Looking back, do you think it's a quality that you are glad you possess?

JAMES: Oh yes. Yes, I am glad I possess it. I think it saves me from much messiness, much messiness of human relationships. It saves me from humiliation, from a lot of distress. But I'm also aware that when I say that it does suggest that I'm too much of a spectator of life and not enough a participant. This may be necessary for me as a writer. But I think it is a danger.

CLARE: What about loneliness? A sense of detachment implies a sense of being apart.

JAMES: I've never been lonely. I've never known loneliness. I like being alone. I have all my life liked being alone. Certainly when I was an adolescent I'd like to go out walking on my own. It's easy for me to say that because I have been lucky in family and grandchildren and friends. I don't ever have to be alone. I sometimes ask myself whether if I had to be alone whether I would be able to bear it with such equanimity. Now, privacy, silence, solitude is immensely important to me.

CLARE: It's rare in a P. D. James book to come across characters who are not in one way or another rather independent or lonely, not part of a very close relationship. Both your central characters in their own ways, Dalgliesh, Cordelia Gray, avoid 'the messiness' in a way.

JAMES: Don't they. They do avoid the messiness. In fact I think Dalgliesh is a man who would admit this, that he uses his job actually as one way of avoiding commitment. He doesn't have to be committed. The hours are difficult, and anyway it's not safe to be committed and when you're investigating murder, you mustn't be committed to the suspect. You have to have some detachment – which you as a doctor must have to have. Otherwise you can't function.

CLARE: Did you ever think of remarrying?

JAMES: No. I didn't and I haven't. I suppose there's an element here of luck. People who have asked me I haven't wanted to marry at all. And I'm glad in fact I didn't.

CLARE: You could have?

JAMES: Yes. I could have. Yes. I haven't wanted to. I think you know that this perhaps is one aspect of selfishness, especially if you like living alone. If you do live alone and you're a writer you have life so much on your own terms. You need to have a great affection and respect for someone in fact to want to share life with that person. In youth, one is looking for a father for one's children, looking for a sexual relationship, looking for all sorts of things. In old age, one is looking, if one is looking at all, for something rather different. I am aware that someone living alone can live a selfish life and this is something that I have to guard against.

CLARE: You make the life of a writer, the task of a writer very central. When I ask you about death you say how many books you have left to write if you live to seventy-five. If I ask about detachment you say 'Well the detachment has helped me being a writer.' If I ask you about regrets you say, 'Well I wish I'd started earlier because I would have written more books.' And if I ask what are the advantages of the detachment, because I'm very aware of the disadvantages, you say, 'Well, it was bound up with being a writer.' What do you make of it?

JAMES: Well, this is really very difficult. Because you see part of me rather resents the writing, because there are so many things I like doing. I mean I have a strong streak of indolence. I quite like doing nothing. I like fuddling round bookshops and antique markets. I like going and visiting my friends. I love going and visiting my children and grandchildren.

CLARE: You don't have to write.

JAMES: Exactly – I don't have to.

CLARE: You're known. You've made your name. If you said to the world 'That's it, I've done it' you wouldn't have to go on doing it.

JAMES: No. My younger daughter said to me 'We all know you're a clever lady now, Mummy – stop it.'

CLARE: What did you say to her?

JAMES: Well. I think this is why I seem to lay so much emphasis on it. It's not that I think I'm a great writer. I know I'm not a great writer, but I do need to do it. I resent this need somewhat because there are so many other things I do enjoy doing. This probably accounts for the fact that my books take up a very long time to write. I don't produce a book a year. I'm not very disciplined, but I do seem to need to do it.

CLARE: And if you didn't do it. What do you think would happen?

JAMES: If I didn't do it now, not very much really. In fact I'd probably have a rather jolly time really, doing all the other things that I rather want to do. Though maybe in two years I'd start getting a little broody, and feel restless and want to get started again. In the past when I was younger, before I had a body of work behnd me, if someone had said you are not going to write another book, this is very difficult for me to visualise. Very difficult. I think this would have caused some fairly deep-seated unhappiness.

CLARE: You started writing when your husband was already ill.

JAMES: Yes. I mean I knew from a very early age that I was a writer.

CLARE: You did.

JAMES: Certainly from early childhood I knew I was a writer. I was a very late starter for a number of reasons, and indolence was certainly one of them, but also there was the need to qualify in a profession that would support my children and my husband. When I was in the Health Service I used to go to evening classes and got a diploma in Hospital Administration and a diploma in Hospital Records. It was the kind of job where a woman had to be better qualified than a man in order to get any kind of senior post and it was necessary for me to get a senior post. So I was a late starter. I can remember – it is a story I told before but it was very, very seminal – the moment when I realised that there never was going to be a convenient time and if I didn't get started I would not be a writer, I would be saying to the grandchildren 'Of course I always wanted to be a novelist.' And this really physically brought a sense almost of horror you know that this really was a possibility and I can remember at the time thinking, 'Well this is intolerable.' So I began to make an effort, and got the first book written.

CLARE: One last question. You've described how a sense of order is important, how indeed the story that you write while it is all about the disturbance of order, at the end at least order to some extent is restored. You are yourself a very ordered individual. You value control. It's an organised life being a writer. It calls for a sense of discipline. I think you value order in society. There is more than a hint of regret that our society is rather disorganised. Have you ever in your life felt that you were teetering on the brink of being out of control? Have you ever been out of control in your life?

JAMES: I can remember one occasion when I was on holiday from a job and my mother-in-law was ill in bed. My husband was ill and the children were home from boarding school. We were a doctor's general practice house and I was trying to cope with it. And I got I suppose desperately over-tired and I did have a feeling that somehow I was losing control, that I just wanted to do something that would mean people would come along with an ambulance and take me off and get me out of it. It was only that one occasion and I must say it was very frightening and it did give me an insight into how people must feel, particularly women whose lives are just too much for them – that sense that I can't do this, I can't cope another minute and if I go mad that will settle it very nicely. And maybe some of them found that way out, and some of them have physical illness and some of them maybe express violence against what they see as the source of their problems. But that of course was a very minor and fairly temporary difficulty for me. I never otherwise remember being out of control. I can remember throughout my life certainly being anxious. I suspect that perhaps writing the kind of books that I do is one way in which I do deal both with subconscious aggression and with anxiety.

Derek Jarman

I interviewed Derek Jarman in 1990. Four years earlier, he had discovered that he was HIV positive. The recording of the interview, initially scheduled for a day in April, had to be postponed. He was still recovering from a chest infection which had necessitated admission to St Mary's Hospital and which, straight-forwardly and with not a hint of self-pity, he describes in the interview which, eventually, took place on 29 June 1990. In a diary, which he published in 1991 entitled *Modern Nature*, he wonders whether the relapse (which may or may not have been HIV-related) had been triggered by a letter from his Aunt Moyra which described in some detail his father's extremely violent behaviour. Not merely did father and son have distressing battles over food – his aunt confirmed that his father would try and force-feed the protesting, defiant four-year-old – but on one dreadful occasion his father threw him out the window in front of his horrified, screaming mother. Hardly surprising, therefore, that much of the content of the interview concerns his father or that, until a couple of months earlier, he had 'buried all of this'.

AIDS, homosexuality, childhood, film-making, death are the themes of this interview. His was and remains one of the most stark, clear, unequivocal voices in the AIDS debate. With me he is characteristically frank about his earlier promiscuity, about his decision to have a HIV test, about his subsesquent celibate behaviour (although one or two things he has said since suggest that this has sadly changed). Even in 1990, when the public debate about AIDS was well under way, not too many people were prepared to discuss their own sexual activities, attitudes, practices in much detail if indeed at all. The eighties had seen the emergence of AIDS as a deadly, previously unknown and untreatable disease. The bland assumption that modern medicine had tabulated all the known diseases and was well on its way to taming them had been well and truly shattered. Through the decade the obituary columns were increasingly filled by young, previously healthy, sexually active individuals, overwhelmingly male, who had sickened and died of the disease.

While the issues of death and dying are universal, the necessity of facing the fact that large numbers of young people are dying in their prime from a communicable disease which we are unable to treat is, for the generations living now, completely new. For anything comparable we have to return to the epidemics of tuberculosis at the end of the nineteenth century and the first half of the twentieth century. So how does someone who learns that he is HIV positive actually cope? When in the middle of winter he gets a temperature which may signal a trivial influenza but may be a potentially lethal pneumonia, a harbinger of death, what does he do?

AIDS is a disease of socially disenfranchised groups. It is circumscribed by stigma and prejudice. It is not of course unique in this regard. An illness with which I am professionally familiar, schizophrenia, is similarly regarded. Few who suffer from it are in a position to describe what it is like and how they cope. Fortunate in this respect are the sufferers from AIDS for there are those like Derek Jarman who can powerfully articulate their feelings and preoccupations, who can energetically campaign for greater public information and education, who can tirelessly lobby for better facilities and treatment.

Derek Jarman's discussion of the changes at that time in his sexual behaviour makes interesting reading. His experience is in line with some of the early findings of changes in sexual behaviour reported in studies of homosexuals in San Francisco. Those men who continued to engage in high-risk sexual behaviour tended to be those who did not believe in AIDS or did not believe it could be spread sexually. Such men, numerous in the mid-1980s, appear, thankfully, to be much less evident today. Secondly, many homosexuals who did believe in AIDS and its sexual transmission had not changed their sexual behaviour because to do so would mean that they would be ostracised and alienated in their community. As the Director of the AIDS Health Project at the University of California (San

Francisco), James W. Dilley put it, 'High-risk sexual behaviour was felt to be an expected and necessary activity if one were to be accepted by one's peers.'[1] Then there were those homosexuals who felt they just could not make the changes necessary, they just did not have the skill or capacity to discuss a potential sexual encounter and place limits on the behaviour that would take place. Such men felt helpless and largely at the mercy of their sexual impulses and those of any partner.

Derek Jarman, as he makes plain in the interview, decided to take a test for HIV, assessed the positive result and concluded what he had to do. Given his personality and intelligence, there is no question of ambiguity on his part concerning the status of AIDS. It is a dangerous disease and it is sexually transmitted. He clearly is a man who sees himself in control yet wise enough to recognise that for none of us is control absolute. I was, for example, conscious that in assuring me that 'even safer sex could go wrong and that if one really was in love with someone one had to remain celibate' he was also struggling to persuade himself of such a purist strategy. Why did I not point this out? I don't know – perhaps time, I think I was more concerned at that moment with his possible guilt about the past then his struggles in the future. But a reassurance I commonly, and perhaps self-deceivingly, fall back on when confronted as I often am with evidence from an interview of an observation missed or a road not taken, is that the listener can and often will make the connection I have missed or muse on the question I have not asked. Sadly, the constraints of a single interview conducted over a couple of hours at most ensure that much more is left unsaid than can be said, unasked than can be asked.

The psychiatric perspective on homosexuality remains an uneasy one. It is less than twenty years since the Board of Trustees of the American Psychiatric Association, after a debate marked by rancour and acrimony, decided to remove homosex-

[1] J. W. Dilley (1983) Psychiatric sequelae of HIV. In *Aids: Psychiatric and Social Perspectives*. Edited by L. Paine, Croom Helm, Beckenham, Kent

uality from the *Diagnostic and Statistical Manual of Psychiatric Disorders*, its official list of psychiatric disorders. Some psychiatrists, infuriated by an action which they believed had been hurriedly taken in reponse to pressure and threats by Gay Liberation groups, forced a referendum involving the full membership of the American Psychiatric Association and aimed at reversing the decision and restoring the disease status of homosexuality. One particularly vigorous proponent of the view of homosexuality as psychopathology was the psychoanalyst Charles Socarides. In his book, *The Overt Homosexual*, published in 1968, Socarides argued that:

> Homosexuality is based on the fear of the mother, the aggressive attack against the father, and is filled with aggression, destruction and self-deceit. It is a masquerade of life in which certain psychic energies are neutralized and held in a somewhat quiescent state. However, the unconscious manifestations of hate, destructiveness, incest and fear are always threatening to break through.[1]

Socarides, in common with many psychiatrists who insist that homosexuality is a pathological condition and one linked with other psychopathologies including manic depression, schizophrenia, paranoia and severe personality disorder, insisted that the effort to find love, stability and security in a homosexual relationship is doomed, not because of society's hostility but because of the intrinsic disturbance at the heart of the condition.

In 1974, nearly 11,000 American psychiatrists solemnly voted on whether homosexuality was or was not a disease. Critics of orthodox psychiatry, such as R. D. Laing and Thomas Szasz, declared that a more concrete example of the extent to which psychiatry crucially differs from the rest of medicine would be hard to find. Just imagine asking endocrinologists to vote on whether diabetes is a disease, they mocked. In the

[1] C. Socarides (1968) *The Overt Homosexual* Crune & Stratton, New York

event, 58 per cent voted in favour of dropping homosexuality from the disease classification while 37 per cent voted in favour of continuing to regard it as psychopathology.

Fear of the mother, over-identification with the mother, an absent, weak father, a harsh, punitive, rejecting father, a mixture of these stereotypes are amongst the plethora of parental characteristics, infantile experiences and family dynamics which have been put forward with varying degrees of conviction to 'explain' the genesis of homosexuality. For Freud homosexuality was a natural feature of human psycho-sexuality, a stage through which most people pass on the way to full sexual maturity but at which some are blocked or arrested. Classical Freudian theory, therefore, envisaged homo-sexuality as an instinctual fixation at a stage short of 'normal' heterosexuality. But why did such an 'arrest' happen? At first Freud thought that male infants destined to become homosex-uals manifested an excessive inborn interest in their own genitals. Subsequently he was to suggest that homosexuality was linked to the profound frustration experienced during the oedipal phase by those boys who had developed especially intense attachments to their mothers and whose frustration turned them away from the female as an object of sexual satisfaction and to the male. Then the theoretical explanations became even more complicated.

There were cases, Freud argued, where the intense attach-ment to the mother was transformed into a wish to enjoy sex in the way she did. As a consequence, the father becomes the object of love and the individual strives to submit to him as the mother does, in a passive-receptive fashion. Alternatively fear of the anger aroused in the father by the son's oedipal desires for his mother could result in the young boy withdrawing from his attachment to his mother and thereafter only a homosexual attachment to men would provide sexual gratification without anxiety about castration.

Freud in his attempt to identify the roots of homosexuality concluded that this retarded stage of sexual development was the result of a series of combinations of inherited, constitutional and environmental influences. To an extent which is quite modern, he attempted to occupy the middle ground between biology and environment. Whatever the wisdom of regarding homosexuality as some form of immature sexual development, what does appear justified even now is Freud's pessimism that anything could be done to alter a homosexual's sexual orientation and nearly a century of therapeutic strategies involving everything from classical psychoanalysis to drug therapy, from counter-conditioning to prayer bears him out.

In the course of a 'Letter to an American Mother', written in 1935, Freud wrote:

Dear Mrs —
I gather from your letter that your son is a homosexual. I am most impressed by the fact that you do not mention this term yourself in your information about him. May I question you, why you avoid it? Homosexuality is assuredly no advantage but it is nothing to be ashamed of, no vice, no degradation, it cannot be classified as an illness; we consider it to be a variation of the sexual function produced by a certain arrest of sexual development. Many highly respectable individuals of ancient and modern times have been homosexuals, several of the greatest men among them (Plato, Michelangelo, Leonardo da Vinci etc.). It is a great injustice to persecute homosexuality as a crime, and cruelty too. If you do not believe me, read the books of Havelock Ellis.

By asking me if I can help, you mean, I suppose, if I can abolish homosexuality and make normal heterosexuality take its place. The answer is, in a general way, we cannot promise to achieve it . . .

Subsequently, psychoanalysts such as Sandor Rado, Irving Bieber and Charles Socarides were to replace such Freudian pessimism with a vigorous therapeutic enthusiasm, insisting that homosexuals could be treated and 'cured'. Therapy would focus on the uncovering of the unconscious desire to achieve masculinity, on the analysis of oedipal fear of incest and aggression, on the supposed discovery of the role of the penis as a substitute for the mother's breast, on the surfacing of the yearning for the father's love and protection, on the recognition of the presence of repeatedly suppressed heterosexual interests and desires. Therapy would focus on any and all of these and therapy would, for the most part, be singularly ineffective. Today, the wheel has turned again and the prevailing orthodoxy is that homosexuality is a minority sexual preference, probably biological in origin but with some contribution from environmental factors such as early upbringing and family dynamics. Thirty years on from the Wolfenden Report which ridiculed the claims for the disease status of homosexuality, nearly twenty years on from the landmark decision of American psychiatrists, the argument still rages.

Psychiatry, with its language of immaturity, fixation, developmental arrest, still seems evasive on the subject of homosexuality. Derek Jarman's own account of his homosexuality, like every individual account, challenges the global, impersonal, academic assumptions about homosexuals and homosexuality. It is a testimony of passionate commitment, creative energy, personal involvement. Whether talking about his tortured, broken, despairing father, his pastoral, therapeutic garden, his disease and impending mortality, Jarman's is the voice of sanity and common sense.

CLARE: Derek Jarman was born on January 31st 1942. His father, a New Zealander, was an RAF pilot during the Second World War. After boarding school, Derek took a general degree at King's College, London, became interested in painting and architecture and studied art at The Slade. His interest took him into cinema and theatrical design and then into film-making and his films include *Sebastian, Jubilee, The Tempest, Imagining October* and *The Last of England.* He has received distinguished awards abroad, including the Los Angeles Film Critics Award in 1988. In 1986 Derek Jarman learned that he was HIV positive. Derek Jarman, is there any particular reason that you agreed to be interviewed in the psychiatrist's chair?

JARMAN: I think partly a sort of vanity and I wondered where the limits were, do you know what I mean, and I thought that you might be able to put me through it so there was a moment when I said enough, enough Anthony. I think that's probably the major reason. Curiosity I think.

CLARE: Are you naturally curious about yourself?

JARMAN: I think I am. I think that a lot of my work has been autobiographical and I've written books which are autobiographical so I am interested in myself, yes.

CLARE: When you look at yourself, are you struck by your past? Does it seem an unusual one to you?

JARMAN: Yes it does, in some ways. I mean I think it's a past which was very much made by pressures, external pressures. I'm not certain it was a past I would have expected when I was much younger, say when I was at school.

CLARE: The striking features being? What is it when you look at it that makes you say that?

JARMAN: Well, I think the first thing was that in the late fifties, you know, when I left school the realisation that I was homosexual was a great problem because there was no information around at that time for people to actually evaluate this situation and one really, for several years, thought one was probably the wickedest person in the world and probably the only one like this. One's information came through the tabloids of 1950s, trials and things.

CLARE: You discovered it when? You were born in 1942. What age did you realise that you were homosexual?

JARMAN: I don't really know. It's very difficult to actually tell. But I think I must have known in my early teens, but there were no words for anything so it was very difficult to actually formulate any real ideas about this. I mean one was actually quite lost.

CLARE: Some people, as you know, hearing that you're homosexual will be speculating on the various influences and doubtless we'll return to that. But in terms of when you did realise without really any doubt that you were a homosexual, when would that have been?

JARMAN: Somewhere towards my seventeenth birthday I should think really.

CLARE: That's 1959.

JARMAN: Yes, about 1959. As for the whole Nurture and Nature debate, I think one is born that way really.

CLARE: You do?

JARMAN: Yes.

CLARE: Any particular reason that you say that?

JARMAN: I don't know. It's something I feel in my bones, because otherwise one falls into the whole area of criticism, of proselytising and all of this sort of area and I don't really believe that's true.

CLARE: And in your experience, let's talk about you, yourself, there was no particular influence? For instance, during the time you were at school? What kind of school was it?

JARMAN: Well, it was a boarding school, but in my particular area there was no sex involved, as it were. I think people think of English boarding schools as a hive of sexuality, but actually there was one boy, who was expelled for sending a love letter to someone else, so I think that's about as far as he got.

CLARE: And your own background, what sort of person was your father?

JARMAN: My father was, in some ways, a very admirable person and also very difficult. I had a very difficult relationship with my father but I don't believe this again tells one anything about one's sexuality. I think he himself was under great stress, you know. He was a pathfinder towards the end of the war and ran bombing missions all the way through the war and I think the moment that I started to talk he thought I should behave rationally. And he came back presumably very tired from these bombing missions and he found this naughty child there.

CLARE: He would come back from the war, you noticed this after the war?

JARMAN: Well I don't know, that is all supposition. It's extremely difficult to know but I wouldn't eat and obviously with rations and you know the way they were, my mother

would cook up presumably the only egg that w̶
house that day for me and I would turn it down, anᵈ
to drive my father absolutely wild and it would end u̶
him attempting to force-feed me. And then real battles of
course, me screaming and being sick and my mother not
knowing what to do and I found out this actually in detail
only about a few months ago. I got into contact with a long-
lost aunt and I asked her, do you know what I mean, what
had been happening when I was four, because I'd actually
buried all of this. I knew the relationships weren't hot and I
suddenly became aware of why I spent all these holidays
with my grandmother, because the family had decided to get
me away from him so that there was sort of quiet.

CLARE: And she told you this.

JARMAN: Yes, she told me this. I mean my father wasn't loved
by the rest of the family, he was loved by my mother but
both my grandmother and all of the brothers and sisters
disliked him immensely.

CLARE: Because they saw him as?

JARMAN: I don't know, I mean I think the treatment he meted
out to me when I was younger was the thing that actually
upset them so much.

CLARE: Were you specifically the target. Did you have brothers,
sisters?

JARMAN: I've a sister.

CLARE: Older? Younger?

JARMAN: No, she's younger but I think she in a way didn't
become a target until she was you know twelve or thirteen,
but it was always the eldest boy, I mean in a sense it was me
and then my sister's eldest son so it was something which
actually went through another generation.

CLARE: Did you get any sense of what it was he wanted?

JARMAN: I don't know. I think at the end he was extremely
lonely. I think the whole business of running these bombing missions in the war, a sense of, a huge sense of loss
and it was quite unbridgeable. It was a very difficult relationship. And also for my sister because as he grew older he
became a kleptomaniac. Actually the first thing that ever

disappeared was my mother's engagement ring and then various things disappeared and it wasn't until after my mother died that we realised that he was the one who was taking it, after his eldest grandson actually accused him of stealing a watch.

CLARE: And when he died, did you find all this stuff?

JARMAN: Well, we did! It was extremely difficult, we discovered a house with really sort of mad collections of things like baked-bean tins or, you know, a collection of lavatory paper which would last for a lifetime, and then objects which we didn't know what to do with, it was very difficult. We rang up his nearest friends down in Lymington and asked them whether they had lost things and actually most people seemed to know about it. And my sister had, in the meantime, been to see the RAF because, you know, they have a department of psychiatry and they'd said there was very little they could do, he was seventy, in his seventies, and we just had to live with it. This was not in any way an unusual situation. But it was a difficult thing for a family to cope with, particularly, I think, for my sister more than myself.

CLARE: Were you frightened of him?

JARMAN: Yes, I think I probably was at times.

CLARE: Was he a large man?

JARMAN: No, he wasn't, he was the same size as I am, he was sort of about five foot eleven.

CLARE: That's large enough for a four-year-old boy. And your mother, throughout all of his, how did she cope?

JARMAN: She was very much in love with my father. I think that the whole marriage had been opposed by my grandparents slightly but she'd won her way in this very middle-class suburban household. You've got to think back to before the war and my aunt said, 'Well, she had only, you know, one boyfriend and then she met your father so she'd led a very sheltered life.'

CLARE: What sort of relationship did you have with her?

JARMAN: It's very difficult to know. The whole thing again was overshadowed by illness because my mother developed breast cancer in her early forties and was at the time given rather a short time to live. Any sort of teenage revolt or fighting disappeared at that point in order to spare her and in fact she lived for another eighteen years or so. So we lived in this sort of suspended state. I mean most kids have flaming rows presumably with their parents at the age of fourteen or fifteen or so. We just didn't do that, my sister or myself. We actually buried this. And my mother was very selfless during this illness which nowadays I wonder about because at the time I thought it was very admirable, but I'm not so certain it wasn't again the pressures of suburban life which made her this way and I wish, having been ill myself, she had sort of said, 'I'm not really feeling up to cooking lunch, why don't you go and get some fish and chips,' or something.

CLARE: Because in fact she battled on.

JARMAN: She battled on.

CLARE: Were you conscious of that kind of martyrdom?

JARMAN: Yes, I was.

CLARE: So what did you do with your negative feelings, difficult if she's battling so selflessly, what do you do with yours?

JARMAN: Yes. I think I was very lucky, I always had my work, you know, so my work became the centre of my life really. Eventually it became film, but it started off as painting. That was an area I was able to inhabit.

CLARE: With things like your anger?

JARMAN: It fuelled work and it always upset me of course, I mean a lot of my films have been fuelled by moments of anger and I still fizz with anger at moments. I can go quite blank. It's usually sort of self-inflicted anger. I doesn't usually spill out to other people. It's just anger at the world in general and I find myself literally pacing round a room and sort of shouting inside really.

CLARE: What sort of things would provoke it?

JARMAN: Oh, I don't know, they're usually sort of political situations, all the problems when one sees, say, reporting about, I don't know, some sort of homosexual murder or something like this, and sort of unforgiving things from the Church, Section 28 on homosexuality made me pretty cross.

CLARE: And you would physically . . .

JARMAN: I physically fizz and I physcially would be upset with myself for fizzing as well because I would sometimes say I don't think this is the best, I could see that some of the films, particularly say *The Last of England*, were fuelled by this and, and I stepped back at the end and said to myself, 'Is it a good idea that work should be fuelled by anger?' But I think a little anger is necessary to fuel work as well.

CLARE: Given what we said about the possible ways in which homosexuality emerges, the great genes versus environment issue, you know well that people focus on the relationship between the homosexual and his mother, the homosexual and his father. What do you make of the fact that in that sense your family dynamic seems to fit the bill?

JARMAN: My family dynamic does fit the bill but I'm certain that that is not the reason because one of the things that I've often done in my life is ask people what is your relationship with your parents and, yes, in many cases the strong mother and the absent father if you like, the weak father if you like, comes up, but I don't think it's actually in any way universal.

CLARE: Or significant?

JARMAN: I think it's of interest, but I mean it's rather like the debate on the HIV thing, you know, does lifestyle play any part in this? Well maybe if you smoke like a chimney, yes it does, this would predispose you to illness. On the other hand people can smoke like a chimney and be OK.

CLARE: And don't get the virus. What about the way in which it developed? Did you ever have a heterosexual relationship?

JARMAN: No, not in the full sense, in the sexual sense, no. But I mean it's very difficult to know where sexuality impinges on this, but most of my relationships with other men have not actually been based on sex.

CLARE: But do you think that's one of those misunderstandings that people have, they tend to see homosexuals as having relationships that are always sexual with other men?

JARMAN: Yes I think they made a terrible mistake there. I think it's again partly because an awful lot of homosexuals aren't visible and live in absolutely stable relationships all of their lives. They don't really fit media criteria, but I don't really believe that they are in any way different to heterosexuals. It's always quite funny, it's usually the heterosexuals who are boasting about their conquests who are the ones who are most prescriptive about telling us that homosexuals lead promiscuous lives.

CLARE: Did you?

JARMAN: I think I did, but it was part and parcel of a revolt that was against the past and those prescriptions that occurred in the seventies. I was celibate until I was about twenty-two and in fact until my late twenties I had very few sexual encounters and I think at twenty-two I might have been horrified at myself at thirty-two. I was a very serious young man listening to Gregorian chant and things like this. I think this is partly a reaction to, you know, the problems that I had looking back on it.

CLARE: Did going to the United States make a difference? You spent some time in San Francisco in North America.

JARMAN: Yes, the States was always a sort of Shangri-La. I mean you know a lot of younger artists went to America, partly I think for their work but also for freer sexual mores there.

CLARE: And you did?

JARMAN: I went on holidays but I never stayed there, I always came back. I nearly stayed in the early seventies which was the time where my life, as it were, was perhaps the wildest and then I decided, I think it was partly self-preservation, to come back to England.

CLARE: How wild was it?

JARMAN: I don't really know, it probably wasn't wild at all, but it seemed wild to me, I mean I was out pretty well every night, and there were drugs involved in it of course in the late sixties and seventies.

CLARE: Nowadays we're preoccupied, and we'll come back to it, with AIDS. But in those days what about the problems of VD?

JARMAN: Well, it was very prevalent.

CLARE: I mean would you have contracted it?

JARMAN: Oh yes, I did.

CLARE: A number of times?

JARMAN: Yes, I did, both gonorrhoea and I actually had syphilis once.

CLARE: Did it scare you?

JARMAN: No not any longer because the doctors didn't seem to be scared by it.

CLARE: Were you involved in any long-standing, by that I mean a particular relationship that would have lasted some years?

JARMAN: Yes, at the moment I'm involved in the relationship of my life in fact.

CLARE: How long have you been involved?

JARMAN: Well, only three years but so long as my life goes on this one will last, I know but it's taken a long time to find someone.

CLARE: Do you think, and again these are subjective judgements I realise that, but your opinion is in this instance as valuable and more valuable than most, do you think it is more difficult for a homosexual to find that kind of supportive, stable, long-lasting relationship?

JARMAN: It wouldn't be if the pressures of society were removed but they are so strong and it's so difficult, there's no legally binding situation for us and appalling things have happened in the last few years when some people who've been living together maybe for twenty years and one of them has died suddenly and they're not next of kin or anything and they have no right to really be even at the death bed, you know, and the family can come along and have them removed. While there is no legal or other structure in which these relationships can flourish like anyone else's, this is bound to happen. The pressures are so enormous. I think things have changed of course in the last twenty years and I think on the whole they've slowly changed for the better. We would never have had a conversation like this, I mean twenty years ago it would have been impossible. The fact that we can have a conversation as open as this is part and parcel of this change and so things have improved.

CLARE: When did you become aware that there was a disease called AIDS?

JARMAN: It's very difficult, I suppose some time in about '82 or '83.

CLARE: Do you remember how you became aware?

JARMAN: There was just this rumour going around, that people had come down with the kaposi cancer and had mostly been gay men in New York, but it was something that had happened in America at that stage and it took a long time for anyone really to be alerted. I think everyone, including myself, didn't really want to believe this was happening and if you didn't see it happening as I didn't because I was living in London and not in New York, to a friend or acquaintance or something, it was easy enough to actually attempt to ignore it. And I think to a greater or lesser extent everyone tried to do that.

CLARE: And then?

JARMAN: And then it caught up with us. I mean that's as simple as that. When was it? In '84 when the HIV virus was discovered, I mean first of all in the Pasteur Institute and then by Dr Robert Gallow and it had two different names for a while, so that was confusing. And it's about that time when, when one realised there may be a causative agent and that it was possible eventually to test for it. At first people were wary of the test because they didn't believe it would be accurate, I think.

CLARE: What about you? How did it affect you personally?

JARMAN: It worried me, I know when I wrote *Dancing Ledge* which was in 1983 I mentioned the whole thing and said that caution is the best approach to this.

CLARE: And your lifestyle in the early eighties, would it have been much the same as it had been in the seventies?

JARMAN: Yes, it was.

CLARE: Many partners, contacts, friends?

JARMAN: Yes, yes.

CLARE: Now when did you have your first test?

JARMAN: Well, what happened was that of course the advice was not to have the test and the advice has always been not to have the test because again pressures on people who were in ordinary jobs and things were enormous and people lost their jobs immediately, so it was a crisis. It wasn't just finding out that it was you who are HIV positive, but it usually entailed in the early days losing your job and all insurance and absolutely everything so . . .

CLARE: So when you say advice . . .

JARMAN: . . . all the advice, including the doctor's advice . . .

CLARE: Yes, I wanted to ask you . . .

JARMAN: . . . the doctor's advice was not to have the test. They told you not to have it because it's not going to make any difference. Act responsibly, you know what to do. It's not going to help to find out.

CLARE: You mean they'd say, change, certainly modify, your behaviour as if you were positive but don't get a test because . . .

JARMAN: Well, everyone should have done that in any case, I mean really that . . .

CLARE: Should have modified their behaviour?

JARMAN: By now, but of course they haven't. But I mean you know even now, and we're talking ten years or eleven years into this, people haven't modified their behaviour. Many people have but a lot of people haven't.

CLARE: So why did you decide to have it, the test?

JARMAN: Well, the reason why I decided was a great friend of mine came over one evening and said that he had the HIV virus and he was body positive and it was very difficult to talk to him. It was as if some wall had gone up, do you know what I mean? I realised all I could do was commiserate and then after it was all over I said to myself now I'm in a situation where I can't lose a job, I'm you know, a film-maker, if this was any other illness like cancer you would go and have a test, I think it would be a sensible thing to do in your particular case. I always preface everything by saying that these were personal decisions and I don't believe my personal decisions are what other people should do, perhaps. But I decided that I wanted to find out and so I went and had a test. I thought there was a good chance that I would have the virus and I was proved right in fact and I was less shocked than the young doctor who told me and it was just before Christmas four years ago.

CLARE: Had you had to wait long between having the test and getting the result?

JARMAN: It was about, I think it was about a week or so, probably ten days.

CLARE: Had you thought much about it while you were waiting?

JARMAN: No, I hadn't. I was quite fatalistic about it. But then when I discovered I had it then the next thing was, or the first advice from the doctor was, to keep it completely secret and I'm afraid I'm not very good at secrets, so I decided that I had to work a way out of actually telling people.

CLARE: And you wanted it public knowledge because?

JARMAN: For myself, because I don't believe in secrecy and I thought it was very important that someone should be open about this, because up to that time, well, no one in this country had really actually admitted to having the virus and you would even get obituaries of quite famous people who you knew and it would never mention this, it would do somersaults to say they hadn't died of AIDS.

CLARE: Did it change you?

JARMAN: Yes, it changed me a lot in ways that it's very difficult still because the time span is so short to really know.

CLARE: You mentioned that the doctor, breaking the news to you, was more upset than you were. What about subsequently, was there a period of kind of matter-of-fact coping and then did it sink in?

JARMAN: I don't know if it's even sunk in yet, it's very difficult to answer that. I'm not quite certain how aware one has to be of something. I think I'm as aware as it's possible to be of my situation.

CLARE: You'd think of it every day.

JARMAN: Not every day no, I didn't actually. Oddly enough I mean after getting it out of my system in a way I thought about it perhaps every third day. Maybe I should have thought about it every day, maybe one should have become more of an activist but I decided I didn't want it to become the centre. I wasn't going to let it take over completely and that, you know, my film and work should still remain the centre. And it did in fact and has done so in that way I'm fortunate. One can create a film which doesn't even have to mention it, although my new film does and the film that I'm going to make, I hope in the next few months, is actually going to be based around my experiences.

CLARE: Well, now what has been your experience of the illness? You were declared HIV positive at the end of 1986.

JARMAN: Yes, it's about 1986, Christmas.

CLARE: And it had an impact but we're not clear quite how.

JARMAN: Well, it's a very odd impact in the sense that you're told you've got a virus but in fact you're exactly the same as you have been. You have aches and pains, you might have flu' or something, it's will-o'-the-wisp really.

CLARE: You hadn't gone for the test because you'd been ill?

JARMAN: No, no.

CLARE: Did it change your sexual behaviour?

JARMAN: Yes completely, that I can actually say one hundred per cent.

CLARE: Can you say . . .

JARMAN: Well yes, I mean it's difficult to say because other people are involved but I can put it in an abstract way. I mean I have been virtually celibate since that time.

CLARE: Although you told me you've a relationship going.

JARMAN: Yes, but I did also tell you that my relationships weren't totally based on sex so, so . . .

CLARE: Now that is, that is . . .

JARMAN: I would like this to have been different, but I made a decision that I wasn't in this particular relationship even going to indulge in what was called safer sex. I decided in my own mind that even safer sex could go wrong and that if one really was in love with someone one had to remain celibate now, for me, again.

CLARE: Do you look back with guilt?

JARMAN: Yes and no, but I mean I know that I'm in exactly the same situation as everyone.

CLARE: When you say yes . . .

JARMAN: We're all . . . well yes in the sense that, looking back on it I wish that I had perhaps been more aware of what was happening in the earlier days, but then if I think back then it wasn't a possibility because no one really knew.

CLARE: Now in fact I want to go back to this issue of HIV positive. You were diagnosed HIV positive at the end of 1986 you were healthy, you felt fine, you'd no particular symptoms. When did that change?

JARMAN: Well, it's very difficult to know. I mean I came back from Poland in February and felt unwell . . .

CLARE: February?

JARMAN: Of this year, 1990 and then, and then I went to St Mary's, you know obviously because that's the first place I go to, this is my hospital to be checked over and initially I thought I'd come back with some stomach bug because I had an upset stomach and a slight temperature. I returned there about a week or so later and my temperature had definitely increased and they, the doctors, quickly put me into the hospital and I was in within a few hours. In fact I didn't even go home, I just sat there and I found myself in bed in St Mary's where during the course of the next few weeks I was tested and it was found that I had TB which I thought, well that's a bit of a relief, and so I got through the TB which took about five weeks and then I got out in April, I suppose, and a few weeks passed and I developed pneumonia. So suddenly I realised, well, this is definitely one of the illnesses which is HIV related and in fact until some several years ago, until the proper treatments were found, was you know often fatal. So now I'm in a situation where

I'm still taking hundreds of pills each day and I'm wondering what the next thing to do would be.

CLARE: When you started to get the symptoms, did you instantly think of AIDS?

JARMAN: No, I still don't think about it because I'm not quite certain where you draw the line. In other words in a certain sense that there's a problem in the whole thing because at what point do you say someone has got AIDS? The virus itself is not enough. How many opportunist infections do you have to have? So I'm not going to admit quite yet that I've crossed the border line, although I'm certain Mark, my doctor at St Mary's, probably thinks I have.

CLARE: Has it changed your mental attitudes in other ways? I mean is death something you think about more or less?

JARMAN: Death doesn't upset me although I'm quite happy being alive, I can assure you. It's nothing I want to encourage, I mean you know I'm enjoying looking after my garden this year and I'd like to be here next year to see it bloom again.

CLARE: But even in the phrase 'and I hope I'll be here next year to see it' suggests that you've, I mean we should all say that, I realise that, but we don't in general, that suggests to me that you've got a more immediate sense of your mortality than perhaps you might have had five or six years ago.

JARMAN: Yes definitely. I'm absolutely keenly aware of my mortality. I mean I could be here this year, next year, you know, another of these illnesses could come along and chop you down at any one moment and they creep up on you very fast. It's amazing how fast they are, you know, one day you're, you're quite well and it takes three or four days then suddenly you've got TB and you're feeling, you know, not at all well.

CLARE: How much experience have you of death? Have many of your friends died?

JARMAN: Many of my friends have died, yes. I mean many of my friends have died of AIDS, too many, probably about fifteen or so. I mean I've actually stopped counting and many of them have been young, very young. In the world I live in, it is epidemic and disastrous. I'm surprised that people aren't shouting even louder about it than they are.

CLARE: Does that make you fizz with anger?

JARMAN: My own mortality again, I don't know, it's a complicated one. I don't know, I watched my mother dying and it's the only death bed I've been at. It didn't seem to be particularly tragic, in fact I was rather pleased when she died.

CLARE: Because?

JARMAN: Because she'd been very ill and it was quite peaceful and I thought it was a very affirmative experience. So that doesn't worry me in any way.

CLARE: What about your father's death?

JARMAN: My father's death was actually one where my sister and I still wonder whether we did the right thing or the wrong thing. My father died late one afternoon or early one evening when we were down packing up his house and we went and we did not stay with him, either of us. Should we have left? This has become an endless conversation between us.

CLARE: Why did you leave?

JARMAN: I just wanted to get out of it, I couldn't, I couldn't bear it any longer. It was the sadness, I still think about it quite a lot. I think we both do. Funnily enough we think more of him, he's remained a shadow after his death more than our mother, we don't really think about her, I don't think, but quite often when I speak to my sister he still comes up. I mean, is there anything we could have done, did we do it right, you know, I mean all of these things.

CLARE: What would you have liked to have been able to do?

JARMAN: I think it would have been nice to have been able to find some ground at some point towards the end of his life, but it wasn't possible. I think with the best will in the world, I mean I think both she and I did try, but he wasn't having any of it. Even at my mother's death bed it was a disaster because he ran away, you see, and I got terribly upset and we, we had to virtually force him back into the hospital really to say goodbye to her. It was my sister and myself who held my mother's hand as she died, not my father.

CLARE: Where was he?

JARMAN: He was in the other room. He couldn't face it.

CLARE: Do you recognise anything of yourself in him?

JARMAN: Oh a lot, a great deal. I resemble him almost more than my mother now at this stage of my life, probably the tone of my voice or something, I see there. I see more of him there than I do of my mother. There's a certain isolation in my life as well which I think is similar to his but I'm not a person who closes the door so easily on people.

CLARE: And your feelings now about him.

JARMAN: I feel now, I mean I look at him really as a historical person. I can see what happened to a particular generation and I can see what happened to my father. I suppose you could sum it up very simply, you know he fought a war and then at the end of it he wondered, I'm certain, what he'd won, 'cos they in fact lost more just fighting any war even if you've got the right on your side, it's still incredibly destructive. And I think that he, after that, that peace was just a long decline you know. Obviously I suppose you must be very, very focused to run those bombing missions and things. As for pleasure in doing it, I don't think so 'cos he would have talked about it.

CLARE: One of the other things I meant to ask you about the impact of the knowledge of HIV upon you was whether it has added any urgency to your work, whether there are things you want to do and you're conscious that you may not have the time.

JARMAN: I don't think so. I thought it might. I don't think the work is that important in the end, you know I think I've done what I could do, but I mean I don't think if I didn't do anything it would be, it would matter particularly. I'm very happy, I'm building this garden at the moment which is my chief joy and delight, as long as I can do that, that's all I really want to do. I never wanted to be a film director or even a film-maker, I just somehow got diverted into it. I hoped it was an area where you could put a few ideas over, but it was extremely difficult because of course the history of the cinema is one of entertainment rather than ideas on the whole. I mean the one nice thing that I can say about the films, this young man came up to me in Glasgow and he said to me, 'Derek,' he said, 'I saw *Sebastian* on the television when I was, I don't know, sixteen,' he said, 'and I had to sort of keep the television almost silent,' he said, 'in case my parents came in,' and he said, 'I didn't understand it,' but he said, 'it changed my life.' I said, 'Oh, that's wonderful, I'm always going to remember that story because when anyone tells me, "Oh Derek you make films that no one understands," all one has to say is, "who cares?"'.

Eartha Kitt

I am often asked how I know whether someone being inter-viewed is telling the truth. I invariably reply how does one ever know? It is the listener who decides, having listened to what is said, how it is said, and what is not said. Listeners who write in very often differ in their interpretations of what they have heard. What is authentic, honest, convincing to one person is bogus, contrived, specious to another. How we come to a judgement that another person is putting it on or saying something for effect is poorly understood. When we make a judgement concerning what some people say about themselves in public we are merely doing what we do all the time in our personal, private lives. Listening to anyone talking, particularly about intimate, personal matters, we are constantly scanning what they see, their tone, attitude, their verbal and non-verbal behaviour. We are more likely to believe someone is telling the 'truth' if what they say fits what we already know of them, how they sound, how plausible their story is when compared to our own experience and so on.

'But how do you know they are telling the truth?' I don't know but I draw my own conclusions and so, as I know from the correspondence generated by the programme, do the listeners. Usually, though not invariably, there is a reasonable degree of unanimity. Listeners are suspicious of anyone who sounds as if they are selling something – a message, a particular view of themselves, a conventionally acceptable package. They are suspicious too of actors, amateur as well as professional. As George Burns is said to have said of acting, 'The secret of acting is being sincere. If you can act that you can act anything.' In this age of the constant interview, with chat show back to back with chat show and newspapers vying with magazines, radio and television to provide the latest in-depth discussion with the great and famous, the professional interviewee has been created. Getting behind the acted interview for something authentic and spontaneous is no easy task.

In the case of Eartha Kitt, this proved something of an understatement! I interviewed her in 1989 when she was performing in London. In the course of a three-hour discussion we consumed a substantial amount of champagne and she gave a tempestuous, high-voltage performance. The details of her life are dramatic enough – told by Eartha Kitt of the gravelly, feline voice and throaty laugh they assume the stuff of a Hollywood epic.

Given her early childhood, it is not surprising that the adult Eartha Kitt is quite frankly suspicious of people – lovers, family, friends. But she also engages in a common psychological defence – she splits the childhood anxiety, self-doubt, fear from the adult competence, talent, composure and gives each an identity, a personality, a name. It is not strictly speaking 'split personality'. Eartha Kitt recognises that Eartha May is not a separate person so much as her alter ego, the poor, shy, abused plantation girl afraid to be alone, the embodiment of traits which she as a public performer must repress, who only comes to life when the spotlights are turned off and the stage vacated. There is no unconscious process at work here, no 'two faces of Eartha'. It is more a case of two sides of the same coin – one private, introspective and insecure, the other public, extroverted and self-confident.

The features of Eartha Kitt's personality include impulsivity and unpredictability, a tendency to develop intense relationships which lead only to disillusion and recrimination. There have been references by others to inappropriate, sudden, intense outbursts of anger, a mercurial temperament. In the interview there are rapid shifts of mood, from exuberance to despondency. The cat-like quality, described by others, exudes a sexual ambivalence – I am sufficiently struck by it to ask her about her appeal to homosexuals. She bats the question back. What do I think? Watching her on stage the night before the interview, I am struck by the ambivalent approach she makes to the men in her audience; at one and the same time she is sensual vamp and reassuring earth mother. She hypes up the feminine – long, slit-to-the-thigh skirts, high heels, outrageous furs, sly references to her reputation as a sex symbol – but exudes an unabashed, raw, masculine power. She is indeed cat-like but it is the lioness and not the domestic pet variety.

Reverberating through what is a difficult interview, full of tangents and abrupt alterations of mood, and indeed through much of Eartha Kitt's life is the theme of rebirth, of a return to a childhood of peace and perfection. The dream of swimming through a tube into a lake and open air where all is beautiful is a fairly straightforward rebirth dream, a transparent wish for a tranquility and stability that were noticeably absent from her own childhood. When her daughter breaks the news of her impending marriage, Eartha wishes the setting was that of an idealised family sitting around an open fire, champagne in hand instead of the more prosaic, dislocated situation – a phone conversation.

But if childhood is agony, brutality, separation, adulthood is full of deceit, betrayal, disloyalty.

The major love affair in her life, involving the millionaire playboy Arthur Loew junior, came to grief over issues of colour, class and who knows what else. Her relationships with men have been consistently unsatisfactory. She remains lonely, disillusioned, hypersensitive. There are hints in the interview that her grim childhood has affected her own mothering skills, the relationship with her own daughter, Kitt. It would be miraculous if it had not.

But my main problem is that the Eartha Kitt story is a great role for a tough, sassy, abrasive woman who stares you boldly in the eye daring you to blink and who responds to any suggestions that she might be aggressive, angry, or just a little touchy with a baleful glare and a throaty growl laden with menace. Eartha Kitt is an actress down to the very toes of her seemingly endless legs. I don't know how much is spontaneous, how much contrived – the quote 'used, accused and abused' I subsequently and repeatedly read in the plethora of interviews she was to give in connection with the launch of her autobiography *I'm Still Here* later that year (1989). 'Nothing in the world is more painful than rejection,' she says and I believe her. 'If your mother gives you away you think everybody in the world is going to give you away.' I believe her once more. The nagging doubt is that these declarations are the stuff of Hollywood movies and Eartha, the consummate actress, is investing the role of interviewee with characteristic energy and intensity.

How do I know if she was telling me the truth? I don't know. What I do know is that sitting in the bare, anonymous basement studio with her was like sitting beside a rumbling volcano. From time to time she erupted. At times, those mesmeric eyes were still, watchful, wary. Throughout there was no time to relax. She talks of surviving and clearly is thinking of herself. It is that kind of self-preoccupation that leads the less observant to deem it selfishness. Yet it is her very insecurity which makes her think of herself so much. She probably does not notice how demanding she can be. Certainly the eyes widen with astonishment when that possibility is put to her.

The tape-recorder switched off, she sets off for an Andrew Lloyd Webber first night. I later hear she slept through the second half. I am relieved to hear it. I too feel exhausted.

CLARE: Eartha May Kitt, singer, dancer, theatre, film, television and recording star, was born on January 26th, 1928 in Colombia, South Carolina, the daughter of a 14-year-old half-black, half-Cherokee Indian girl raped by the white son of a plantation owner. When her mother married an older man, Eartha and her sister were brought up by an aunt in Philadelphia and her career as a singer and dancer began when she joined Katherine Dunham's black dance troupe. She was discovered by Orson Welles in 1951 while singing at a supper club in Paris and became an internationally recognised cabaret star. In 1962 she won the Golden Rose at Montreux and in 1968 was named Woman of the Year by the National Association of Negro Musicians in the US. Her autobiography, *I'm Still Here*, was published in 1990. Eartha Kitt, how do you feel about talking about yourself?

KITT: Scared. Which one of me do you want to talk about?

Which one of me. People want to seemingly talk to Eartha Kitt but nobody wants to talk to Eartha May. She is that ugly duckling that hides under the table all the time with the cats and dogs and the birds. So that's why I say which one of us do you want to talk to?

CLARE: Tell me some of the differences between Eartha May and Eartha Kitt.

KITT: Eartha May is very scared of being seen, she is hiding all the time. Eartha Kitt is the one that says everything's OK, you can talk to me, you can talk to me.

CLARE: She performs.

KITT: Yes she's the one who makes the bread and butter for both of us. Eartha May is the one who's hiding in the woods. She's always hiding. I think some people think that I'm very crazy. I have been treated like a very beautiful person, like the most beautiful woman in the world, the most exciting woman in the world, the most sexy, and men would take me out and they would rather feed me alcohol than give me a meal, particularly in the beginning when I was extremely young and the most beautiful woman in the world, the most exciting woman in the world and all these accolades, but they wanted to take me to bed rather than take care of me, or help me take care of myself. So I don't want to be beautiful anymore. I'm glad that lines are coming in my face, I'm glad that my hair is growing grey and I don't want to be recognised in men's eyes as a beautiful creature anymore. Now I want to be taken care of, I really do. I keep hoping that, through my voice and through my soul and through my spirit that on some record or other, some book that I have written or other, that I can pass it on to my child because I do not want my baby to be suffering what I have gone through. I want her to accept she has to earn her own way too. So everything that I'm doing now, going through, after having gone through all of the men who use me as what you call that, a notch on the belt, (laugh) it's my turn now, really, it's my turn. They treated me like, like a beautiful thing that they wanted to use, abuse and accuse.

CLARE: Given the start you had in life, could it have been any different?

KITT: How can I tell you that, who knows? My mother gave me away and sometimes I think, well it's true, if your mother gives you away you think everybody in the world is going to give you away. I think every man that comes into my life is going to give me away, every contract I make in my path of life is going to sell me down the river and I keep hoping that it doesn't happen again. But I keep trusting, I keep trusting. My mother did not give me away because she was a mean person or she didn't want me. My mother gave me away because she had to. My mother was taken advantage of by the cotton plantation owner's son and I don't know who my father is. I don't even know what tribe I belong to except I do know somewhere along the line that my mother's mother was a Cherokee Indian mother. I got more badly treated from the black kids than I ever did, than I ever gotten treated from the white people. The white people always threw a piece of something, you know, at least they threw me a nut, they threw me something that I could survive on, some seed, something like that. The black people kicked me and put me in a sack, tied me to a tree and whipped my bottom because I was not the right colour, I was not accepted. If you were to ask me what group would you like to belong to, I would have said none, none, I don't want to belong to none of you, I don't want to belong to any of you, I only want to belong to myself.

CLARE: So where is home?

KITT: Home is within me. I may have a house over there or a room over there or a piece of clothing somewhere, but home really is within me, and as long as I do not lose my centre, as long as I do not lose the core of myself, I feel I'm OK and safe. They try though, very often, they try very hard, friends particularly, friends.

CLARE: What do they, what do they do?

KITT: Friends can be your worst enemies because they are the ones who make you feel you can trust them and once you feel comfortable in that relationship, it means you're not watching anymore. Therefore behind your back comes a little something that you were not expecting and it's called a friend.

CLARE: Given that home is inside you and you don't wish to belong . . .

KITT: To a race, creed or colour . . .

CLARE: What about loneliness?

KITT: Loneliness?

CLARE: Have you one or two close friends who've lasted over time?

KITT: Yes.

CLARE: Now how's that come about?

KITT: Because we've proved ourselves to each other through the years.

CLARE: Are you very demanding?

KITT: Not demanding.

CLARE: Testing?

KITT: Testing.

CLARE: When did you discover that you had power, that you by virtue of yourself, caused things to happen around you?

KITT: I don't know if I ever did, I don't think I want to know that.

CLARE: But surely you know it now?

KITT: Not really. Just because the name is the biggest name in the Shaftesbury West End area does not mean that I know I have power because when the lights go out, who's going to pluck it out, any minute it can be plucked out.

CLARE: Yes, that's true, I'm not saying it's a very permanent power, but you know that you exercise over some of these men a certain power?

KITT: Well why do you say men?

CLARE: I suppose men because you've got great sexual power, or so it would seem to me. Are you going to say to me you don't think you have?

KITT: My sexual-ism, if I were to break that word down, sex, OK, S. E. X. Sexuality to me means you fall in bed with somebody and you go with the relationship of the action. Sensuality is something else again.

CLARE: Go on.

KITT: Sensuality. Now if you were to take the word, you can spell it S. E. N. . . . means you have a little sense that you can work with. I didn't think about it before, but now that you're talking about it to me, that's really what I have been doing in so many ways. I have been using my sense in order to use my sensuality in order to make a few cents. I didn't think about that before, I must write that down.

CLARE: Let's take the other power. These are difficult words and you're disciplining me in the use of them and that's no harm. The sensuality is bound up with you as a performer?

KITT: Naturally.

CLARE: I promise we will come back to when the lights go out, but when the lights are on or when the lights turn on what happens to you?

KITT: It's exciting. It's very exciting. It's as though I put on my tribal clothes and I go out and I do my damnedest and I go home and pay my bills hopefully. But when the lights go out I go back into being Eartha May and she's hiding under the floor, she's hiding in the forest and she's with her dogs and her cats and her birds.

CLARE: Now people listening would wonder why hasn't your experience onstage made Eartha May more confident, and less frightened.

KITT: Because I know who I am, I know who I am.

CLARE: And you're really Eartha May.

KITT: That's right.

CLARE: That's when you feel really yourself.

KITT: I feel comfortable there. I do not want, oh my God let me, help me find the words for what I really want to say, because I really want you to understand. I want to be accepted. She wants to be accepted, not really, but you know not really. I'll give you one of these crazy stories about this family that I was given to.

CLARE: As a child . . .

KITT: Yes, I told you, it was a black family and I was used as a Cinderella, you know, working mule, like a horse, like the one who pulls the ploughs and all of that you know. The mother got sick and she wanted to have some medicine, she said I need some medicine and said 'Willie, will you go?' 'No.' 'Gracie, will you go?' 'No.' 'To the white man's store across the forest, through the graveyard, through the St Peter's Church to get the medicine?' And you know being very superstitious, we were brought up with superstition, it's full moon, stuipid me, I said 'I'll go.' But I was not so stupid because I wanted to pay for my reason to exist. So I went and that is Eartha May. Eartha May would have suffered anything in the world in order to say I have a reason to exist. I will earn my own way, so through Eartha Kitt she's doing it. Through the graveyard, through the forest, through the mud, through the hells of Hell, she will do it.

CLARE: When the lights go out do you wish that they would stay on forever?

KITT: No.

CLARE: Why not?

KITT: Because you need the moment to rest.

CLARE: But the sensation, the feelings?

KITT: No, no, even the feeling has to be put to sleep.

CLARE: How much reverberations of that fear as a child are there?

KITT: You mean, am I afraid?

CLARE: From time to time?

KITT: Of course I am.

CLARE: Of what?

KITT: Of not being understood.

CLARE: That worries you a lot. People misunderstand you?

KITT: Even that is not half as fearful as the rejection fear and I don't expect everyone to come into my life and expect to understand.

CLARE: But why do they misunderstand?

KITT: Because there is a difference between Eartha Kitt and Eartha May and they cannot see the difference.

CLARE: You can't cope with that?

KITT: No. Because they see me like I'm sitting here in front of you now. I'm sitting with no make-up. My hair is not done. I did not come to you with the razzamatazz that I present myself with onstage or whatever the character that I am playing. I came to you in plain clothes. My face is absolutely clear and that's how I expect you to accept me. I've no make-up on. I have no eyelashes on. I have no hair-do's.

CLARE: But you are saying to me that many people cannot accept you like that.

KITT: No, of course not. Because they only know the name Eartha Kitt.

CLARE: And that's what they want to see.

KITT: Yes, that's understandable.

CLARE: So what conclusion do they draw when they see you?

KITT: Maybe they expect me to dress up for them. It's like when I'm going jogging or something like that, they say 'My God, is that Eartha Kitt?' I go jogging without any razzama-tazz – I'm myself. You don't expect me jogging through Hyde Park with an Eartha Kitt make-up on.

CLARE: When you're onstage, just pursuing this distinction between the two Earthas, are there times when you're aware of this extraordinary transformation from May to Kitt?

KITT: Yes, very much, very much.

CLARE: If one is very perceptive, would one notice that occasionally Eartha May is there?

KITT: If one is very perceptive.

CLARE: You have an interesting stylistic trick at the end of a tremendously powerful number to mock it slightly, is that a hint?

KITT: Because I'm mocking myself. I have no idea what I'm doing but I also have an idea of what I'm doing. I have no idea of thinking in terms of fornicating the people, because like it has been said 'You can fool some of the people some of the time,' and I don't want to fool any of them any of the time. My heart and soul and my guts and my feet, my legs, my ism is there, but I'm teasing, but at the same time I'm not. In the back of my mind there always seems to be a sense of humour that deals with reality.

CLARE: What about when you came to have a child of your own, and the extent to which that introduces a new reality where you then became not just responsible for Eartha May and Eartha Kitt but there's this new person?

KITT: Yes, it becomes not only a responsibility as far as taking care of someone else is concerned, but it's searching your soul to find out what kind of person you really are, and that's when you can really search inside of yourself to find out whether you are a selfish person or you are a giving person. That's when I realised through my baby and myself I am a very giving person and sometimes very often to a dangerous point. I was going to say not so much to my daughter so much, but even in that area I think so as well, I can be very much over-responsible.

CLARE: In what way?

KITT: Well before I had Kitt for instance I wanted my friends through me to be comfortable because of what the gods have given me. Because of that kind of feeling that I have within myself very often I was taken advantage of. That's why I said to you before friends can be your worst enemies, they don't know when to stop. You give them a finger and they want the whole thing, the whole body and all that. And the same thing I think with a child. I want my daughter to be comfortable but not in such an excessive way that she is no longer using her intelligence. So, as I said, it can be often sometimes dangerous, that you want to be too protective.

CLARE: Have you resolved it?

KITT: I don't think there is any resolving. I think it's up to my daughter to do that. Up to this point I have been very uncomfortable with the idea, the thought, of the empty nest syndrome of my baby being taken away from me. First of all my daughter calls me, I was in Paris, my daughter says 'Mummy,' she calls me up on the phone, 'Mummy, I'm getting married, Mummy sit, sit down Mummy!' I was in the Georges V hotel, I only wished that we had gathered around the fire, something like that you know.

CLARE: Something personal?

KITT: Yes, if they had only sat me down over a candle, over a piece of bread, a glass of wine, my champagne, something like that you know. So I opened up the fridgidaire, took another drink and sat down on the floor by myself. No, it's very interesting because nobody knows what is going on in the heart and soul of someone else, when a trauma comes about. I thought I had prepared myself psychologically and also emotionally for my daughter getting married. It was bound to happen sometime. I expected it. But when it did happen there was a kind of thing like that tradition in a Jewish wedding where one has to stamp on a glass – it was the smattering of my soul, believe me, believe me. Everything went in my soul. He smashed my soul, he smashed my soul. He smashed my heart, he smashed my soul, he smashed my womb, he smashed my guts, he smashed the lot that I brought into this world. I'm empty now, I am very empty now. And my soul is crying and it is not him, it does not matter whom she married, it's not him.

CLARE: Do you dream?

KITT: I dream. Go on.

CLARE: What do you dream about?

KITT: There were three dreams I have had in my whole life that completely give me something to think about because they are constantly repetitive. I keep dreaming about myself in a body of water, in a very plain lake. I am not the world's greatest swimmer but in this dream I seem to be very comfortable in the water. I am trying to take myself from one side of the lake to the other. Then I find myself in a tube – I'm very strong against claustrophobia. For instance, if you put me in a room like this where I cannot see a window . . .

CLARE: This small interview room?

KITT: Yes, if I am in here too long I start to beat against the world. As long as I can see something outside I'm all right. So, I'm in a tube and I have to swim up but the water is very clear. So I'm struggling like a fish, going up very comfortably, and when I get to the other side I just come out in an open lake or pond, whatever you want to call it, and I look out on a very, very very beautiful world – meadows, wonderful trees, fascinating blossoms. Everything is OK. And I just look around and I dive down again, go through the same tube, come out in the same lake that I started in and everything is wonderful. I've had that dream so many times in my life. So do you want to analyse it?

CLARE: When you're in the tube are you panicking?

KITT: No, no, not at all.

CLARE: So there's no sense of unease in this dream? It's a peaceful dream?

KITT: It's a peaceful dream. I think that's how I'm going to die.

CLARE: How?

KITT: Very peacefully.

CLARE: Are you a believer?

KITT: Yes.

CLARE: In something else?

KITT: God.

CLARE: Afterwards? Do you think you would meet people?

KITT: Yes.

CLARE: Afterwards? Do you think you will meet people? Your mother? Want to? What would you ask her?

KITT: I want, no I won't ask her, I will just say to Mummy, 'I understand.' There's nothing to ask.

CLARE: You'd tell her that. Would you meet your father?

KITT: I don't want to know, I do not want to know. At the same time it might be very interesting, I would like to have a battle with him.

CLARE: A battle with him?

KITT: Really, I really would like to have a battle with him, I really would, I really would. How do you men treat us women? You lay down, you pass your seeds on and you leave the woman to do whatever you think it is that the woman should do. You're nomads.

CLARE: Putting this personally, is that what you feared when your daughter married? That's what would happen?

KITT: All right. Let met think about that one. I think I felt that when my daughter married that man would be treating her the way men have treated me and my mother and maybe my mother's mother, all the way down the line.

CLARE: Did you ever meet a man you thought might be different?

KITT: Different from what?

CLARE: From the men you just described, the nomads?

KITT: You mean someone who would not have walked away from me? Arthur Loew.

CLARE: Arthur Loew?

KITT: Yes, yes. I really thought he would never walk away from me. I thought he wanted a relationship, a good relationship. I thought he wanted faithfulness. And I think one of the biggest problems I have, if I was to think of myself in terms of having a problem, is because I'm faithful, I'm a very faithful person.

CLARE: You say it with great passion. They, men, don't sound very likeable or even loveable? Are they?

KITT: Not when they find a beautiful woman whom they want to use, accuse and abuse. They do not think of a woman as being as an intelligent person. They think in terms of a woman as being a beautiful creature whom they can lay down, use, abuse, then accuse and pass their seeds along, whether we want it or not.

CLARE: You said you were superstitious.

KITT: Very.

CLARE: Still?

KITT: Yes.

CLARE: What sort? What sort of superstitions?

KITT: Garlic.

CLARE: Garlic?

KITT: Yes.

CLARE: Tell me about it?

KITT: I eat a lot of garlic.

CLARE: Because?

KITT: Because I think garlic is the one cleanser that I know. Garlic, red pepper, greens, clean my intestines and champagne, providing it's pure, anything that, if you can think of anything of being pure anymore.

CLARE: Have you other superstitions? Other things you have to do before you go on stage, you know the way some people are?

KITT: Once I start putting my make-up on then I'm getting into the character, but with garlic I know garlic will clear my veins.

CLARE: What's it like when you start putting the make-up on?

KITT: I start getting in character. I start changing the character.

CLARE: You sense it.

KITT: Yes.

CLARE: You can actually physically feel it.

KITT: Oh yes, psychologically, you can feel it.

CLARE: Going back to this distinction – Eartha May, Eartha Kitt – in fact as I talk to you, the distinction blurs doesn't it, I mean Eartha Kitt isn't just on stage? Is she? You laugh.

KITT: Both of us are there, mmmn.

CLARE: Very much so, so why do you split yourself like that? Why are they separated?

KITT: Because I'm a very private person, in spite of it, in spite of everything, I'm a very private person.

CLARE: You mean Eartha Kitt is a mask, it covers. Eartha Kitt is very much on show.

KITT: Just a moment, just a moment baby. Every time someone asks me that kind of question it seems to me that I have to give an answer for it, I really do not have an answer for it. I just know when it comes to a time for me to separate myself from the stage personality and Eartha May I do it. I know when it's happening. At the same time sometimes I don't know when it's happening, really.

CLARE: Let me ask you something, because you've said very bluntly, 'I'm changing, the body's ageing but the mind it stays lively and alert.' You, in a sense, are almost saying you embrace ageing, it will, in a sense, release you?

KITT: And maybe that's why I get into trouble all the time, because I'm not interested in remaining physically young, physically young. I only want to be intellectually stimulated, but youth has nothing to do with it. I just want youth to appreciate those of us who have passed through the time span of life in order for us to share something with them, in order for them to say 'I appreciate you.' You know all I'm looking for is a job, really, that's all I want is a job, and as long as my name is the top of the mark, as long as I can put two thousand people, two hundred people, one hundred people, forty people, four, four people, to work.

CLARE: And if it's not top of the mark?

KITT: Somewhere down the line I'm still in there.

CLARE: When I went to see you the other night I was quite struck by the very strong support that you have from the gay community.

KITT: Why do you think that was so?

CLARE: I wasn't clear.

KITT: Well neither am I. But if I was to actually think about it, now that you have put it into this side of my brain, I would think that we're all rejected people, we know what it is to be refused, we know what it is to be oppressed, depressed and then accused. And I am very much of that feeling. Nothing in the world is more painful than rejection. I'm a rejected, oppressed person. That's how I understand them as best I can, even though I'm a heterosexual.

CLARE: Your sexuality doesn't threaten them?

KITT: No, neither does their sexuality threaten me.

CLARE: In this life of yours, have you ever felt that if you didn't wake up tomorrow you wouldn't much care.

KITT: Yes. But I did it anyway.

CLARE: How do you mean?

KITT: Somehow or other I pulled myself together and got there, even though I felt at that particular time ... and the gods were behind me.

CLARE: What is the thing that drives you on? That has driven you on all the way through?

KITT: I would say it's survival.

CLARE: Yes, but that describes what happens. What explains it? What makes it for you worthwhile?

KITT: What makes it all worthwhile, I don't know yet, I really don't know yet.

CLARE: You mean you don't know whether anything makes it worthwhile?

KITT: No, I don't know yet.

CLARE: If you had a wish, that has as yet not been fulfilled, what would it be?

KITT: I would like to be sitting in a meadow, with all my birds and cats and dogs and people around me that I really like and care for and my daughter to come once in a while to visit me. Maybe perhaps that will be my grave.

CLARE: Eartha Kitt, thank you very much.

KITT: And the only thing she'll do is sit on me.

Ronald Laing

On 23 August 1989 Ronald Laing suffered a heart attack on a tennis court in the South of France and died shortly afterwards. Four years before, on the occasion of the publication of the first and only volume of his autobiography, I had introduced him to the audience at a lunch-time talk at the Institute of Contemporary Arts in London. The ICA had asked me if I would and I had accepted although I expressed doubt that Laing would be agreeable. Some years before he had taken offence at a review I had written of his book *The Facts of Life*. I had dubbed it 'boring'. To my surprise, however, he agreed to the ICA proposal and an enjoyable session took place.

He was not in good physical shape at the ICA. He had been drinking heavily and had inexplicably and recently lost a tooth. Nevertheless, he gave a vigorous account of his views on psychiatry, mental illness and the dynamics of the family to an audience, most of whom had not even been born when his first and most original and outstanding book, *The Divided Self*, had been published. I first read the book as a medical student in Dublin in the early 1960s. It made an immense impact on me because of the lucid and convincing way in which it demystified madness, ruptured the divide between the mad and the sane and offered a meaningful explanation of much so-called 'pathological' symptoms and behaviour. In the words of one of his colleagues and supporters, Joe Berke, Laing 'put the person back into the patient'.

In the early 1960s, Ronald Laing undertook extensive research into families at the Tavistock Institute in London. The publication of *Reason and Violence*, which he co-wrote with David Cooper, *The Politics of the Family*, and *Sanity, Madness and the Family* established him as a psychiatrist of repute. The appearance of the extraordinary, poetic work *The Politics of Experience* and *The Bird of Paradise* propelled him to the status of guru. The eruption of student unrest, the growth of the drug culture and the social turbulence in western society related to growing disillusionment with the Vietnam War contributed to the recruitment of Laing to an oddly assorted coalition which met in London in the summer of 1967 as the Congress of the Dialectics of Liberation. Amongst those who spoke were Stokely Carmichael, Gregory Bateson, Herbert Marcuse and Laing himself. A radical view of psychiatry, associated with his name, began to spread around the world. His apocalyptic message shaped and reflected ideas and passions prevalent at this time and contributed to the bracketing of the mentally ill with the criminal, the racial outcast, the sexual deviant and the political dissident in a coalition of oppressed bearers of an authentic statement concerning the human condition.

At the heart of Laingian psychiatry is the belief that much psychotic behaviour is a striving for spiritual enlightenment and transcendence. To the extent that drugs and hospitalisation interfered with such growth Laing opposed them. By the end of the sixties he had moved from the phenomenological analysis of schizophrenic experience to a conspiratorial model of mental illness in which he portrayed the psychotic patient as both a scapegoat driven into madness by hostile malevolent parents and a voyager engaged in a semi-mystical journey of self-exploration, transcendence and growth. Laing spent the early 1970s in Ceylon, the rest of the decade in Britain, where he published four slim volumes, semi-autobiographical, speculative and poetic. The 1980s were unproductive years apart from the appearance of the first volume of his autobiography.

By the time I came to interview him, drugs, drink and a certain degree of Celtic melancholia had taken their toll. Despite the fact that it was early afternoon, Laing was mildly intoxicated when we started and as a consequence much of the interview had to be discarded by my producer. But slowly he sobered up. Given his published views on the nature of family life I was interested in hearing more about his own. His account is incorrigibly bleak — his son, Adrian Laing, who is currently working on his father's biography, tells me that his researches suggest that R. D. Laing somewhat exaggerated the deprivation and bleakness of his early years.[1] Yet Laing talked frankly and movingly about his own depression, his heavy drinking, his philosophical preoccupations.

The interview was well received though there was one surprise that Laing, the fierce critic of the use of drugs in psychiatry, should appear so willing to consider their use should he become seriously depressed. There were comments too about the fact that one of the most depressed subjects to sit in the psychiatrist's chair should have been a psychiatrist.

Shortly afterwards, however, I received a somewhat cryptic letter from R. D. Laing asking me whether I was willing to act as one of his examiners as the General Medical Council was moving to have him removed from the medical register. I wrote back but heard nothing more. While preparing this book I talked with Adrian Laing and he filled me in on the complete story. Some time before the interview a disgruntled patient had complained to the GMC about treatment he had received at the hands of Laing. Eventually he dropped his complaint but the wheels had been set in motion and now the transcript of the interview Laing had with me was included as evidence against him. I am unclear as to quite what in the transcript provoked the move – the most likely explanation lies in Laing's discussion of his drinking and his depression. The GMC, following the procedure laid down for the investigation of complaints against doctors, invited Dr Laing to nominate three psychiatrists who he would agree could examine him. Laing nominated myself, my Irish colleague and Laing's friend, Professor Ivor Browne, and Professor Morris Carstairs, former professor of psychiatry at Edinburgh and a former teacher. Laing insisted that we, in turn, would have to agree to be examined by him and should any tests be required we would have to undergo them too. I never heard whether the psychiatrists nominated by the GMC to examine Laing on their behalf had agreed to these terms. I did!

In the event, Laing agreed to withdraw from the register

---

[1] A. Laing (1992) R. D. Laing, 'The First Five Years'. *Journal of the Society of Existential Analysis* Vol. 2 pp. 24–29.

himself. To practice as a psychotherapist he did not need to be on it. Registration was required only if he wished to practice as a psychiatrist and prescribe drugs. He didn't. Subsequently he spent much of the time in the US. Within four years he was dead.

We are still too close to R. D. Laing's death to be able fully to assess the ultimate worth and impact of his views. His was a powerful voice in the movement to demystify mental illness and he undoubtedly contributed to the process whereby psychiatry moved out of the large, isolated, grim mental hospitals into acute units attached to general hospitals and into the community. His own therapeutic community at Kingsley Hall served as a prototype for many similar non-hospital settings for people in psychological crisis. He challenged the crude reductionism in psychiatry which had followed the enthusiastic introduction of the powerful antidepressant and antipsychotic drugs. He influenced a whole generation of young men and women in their choice of psychiatry as a career.

Of course his extraordinarily powerful Glaswegian rhetoric led to overkill and many relatives struggling to cope with seriously mentally ill patients still find it hard to forgive him for seeming to suggest that they were responsible for the very conditions they attempted to manage. But, as he himself reveals, he had very personal reasons for regarding the bosom of the family with suspicion. He claims to have suffered the ambivalent communications and the mixed messages of distorted domestic life which, as a polemicist, theorist and critic, he was to identify and dissect so vividly in his later professional writings.

In this interview he comes across as a troubled, sensitive, likeable, pugnacious man. I personally am reminded of one of Camus's physicians, those doughty fighters who, despite their own personal afflictions and flaws, refuse to 'bow down to pestilences and strive their utmost to be healers'. In a particular sense, everyone in contemporary psychiatry owes something to R. D. Laing and, whatever the profound shortcomings in his life-long argument about the nature of mental illness, he at all times demanded that the plight of the mentally ill be taken absolutely seriously.

CLARE: Dr Ronald Laing was born in Glasgow in 1927, graduated in medicine in 1951 and entered psychiatry. In 1960 he published his first book *The Divided Self*, which set out to demystify mental illness and to bridge what Laing saw as a gulf between the so-called insane 'them' and the alleged sane 'us.' A succession of books in the sixties on the family, interpersonal communication and schizophrenia reached an enormous audience, and Laingian psychiatry – for his name became attached, though not by him, to a particular school of psychiatry – became associated with the idea of mental illness as a journey, a potential semi-mystical experience, and the mentally ill as in a sense possessed of rare insights. In 1988 he published the first volume of his autobiography *Wisdom, Madness and Folly* subtitled *The Making of a Psychiatrist*. Dr Laing, I was surprised that you agreed to be interviewed by me in this series and I wondered really why?

LAING: Maybe I found the theme of the series a very congenial one, the events and influences in an individual's life which may or may not have exercised a crucial impact on his or her subsequent development. Well I find that theme a very challenging one to consider in my own life and it also raises any number of theoretical and practical problems in our line of business.

CLARE: It takes me back to your background. One of the things that struck me when I read *The Facts of Life* which you published nearly a decade ago I think, is that as you portray your early life, your early years in Glasgow, a picture of you as a solitary only child in a rather bleak and certainly rather pleasureless early home is a very striking image, it comes out of your prose.

LAING: Of course I didn't think of myself in those terms at the time. But the bleakness and unhappiness about it periodically in my life I remember again, some things, and then I repress them. I don't think I've fully recalled and assimilated some of the negative side of that childhood. Some children do separate off their own parents or their family and they're very exceptional. Well I never made that move in my mind so I took the family that I was living in sort of for granted, like every other family. But it wasn't, it took me quite a number of years to realise that. Joe S, who was a neurosurgeon round about the time when I was out of the Army, he said to me 'Don't you realise your mother's mad?' and I was absolutely, I was quite offended (laugh).

CLARE: What struck him about her that made him make that statement?

LAING: Well it's difficult to epitomise. Well I'll tell you a story about my mother. My second eldest daughter, when she was fourteen or fifteen, told me that my mother had told her that she had made herself or acquired a little figurine called Ronnie, Ronald, that she was sticking pins in its heart you know, to give me a heart attack.

CLARE: Your mother was doing this.

LAING: This was, yes, this was what my daughter told me my mother was doing.

CLARE: You were the only son, the only child, and she was about forty when you were born.

LAING: She was about thirty-six.

CLARE: You were the only child.

LAING: The only child, you see they had been married for nine years before I came along.

CLARE: I see, was it ever explained?

LAING: No, well she swore the last time this was ever broached and so did my father to me when I was in my mid-thirties – I took him to a sort of downtown Glasgow restaurant bar which he had never been to in his life and he swore to me, man to man, he had no idea at all how I was conceived. And so did my mother say the same, they absolutely denied that any sexual act of intercourse had taken place at my conception.

CLARE: And there's a picture of enormous pathos in your autobiography of you as a tiny boy with a toy horse and underneath is written a little note which ends 'my mother decided I was getting too fond of it and burned it.'

LAING: That's correct. She didn't believe in me getting attached to anything. After this book was published I sent it to my Aunt Ethel who was in her seventies. She said 'Oh your mother would destroy anything you got attached to, that's why if you remember I never gave you a present, I only gave you half a crown, I gave you money.'

CLARE: How did she relate to your father?

LAING: My mother? Oh well I think it was a total disaster. They certainly never appeared to sleep together. He had a room and my mother and I shared a room but not a bed, there were two beds in one room. Later my father moved to the one sitting room, the third room in the house and turned over to me his room at the back of the house which up till then my mother had always referred to as the dog kennel. Well Aunt Ethel's construction of my mother was that she was burned up with envy and jealousy of everyone and particularly my father. I mean after all he was the principal baritone of the Glasgow University Chapel Choir. You'd never imagine that he was worth anything at all as a singer if you heard any comments that my mother would make about his singing.

CLARE: She's still alive now and while I know there's much more you could have published or I sensed there is, nonetheless even what you've written, what you're even saying now presumably could and does cause great offence. Do you see much of her, she lives in Glasgow?

LAING: I don't see her at all. As far as I know she's cut herself off from all communication through reading or television and the radio.

CLARE: She would have read *The Facts of Life*, ten years ago?

LAING: No, no, she's never read it, she's never read herself, as far as I know, a single word that I've ever written.

CLARE: But people would say things to her?

LAING: Yes, someone told her.

CLARE: What did she make of your fame, in the sixties?

LAING: It made absolutely not the slightest difference to her.

She lives so much outside the world in which fame is applicable. I don't think in the south side of Glasgow where she was living anyone in the street would ever have heard of Dr Laing.

CLARE: But pressing you, I mean there are many mothers who don't understand the reason for their offspring's fame, but take a considerable, indeed even personal enjoyment, indeed even take responsibility for the fame in the first place. But there was none of that with you? You were in many ways a household name in the sixties. People who didn't know much about psychiatry knew about Ronnie Laing. So while there might have been a few tenements in Glasgow that didn't, nonetheless they could have easily known an ebullient mother who was keen to bask in the reflected glory. She wasn't that kind of mother?

LAING: Oh, no, no, she didn't see anyone. I don't remember her ever having had a single friend, man or woman. I don't remember anyone ever coming to the house to have tea with her at her invitation. I mean it was a major thing if she entered someone's door.

CLARE: You reveal in this autobiography that you've just written that one of the examples in an earlier book about a boy of seven falsely accused of stealing a pen, which illustrates in that book the double-bind communication – the way in which you're put into a position where whatever you do you invalidate yourself and in some sense confirms something about yourself which is untrue or inaccurate – that turned out to be actually an account from your own background. I wonder the extent to which your own vision of the way humans communicate with each other has borrowed heavily from what sounds, as you describe it, a most remarkable interaction in the Laing family back in Glasgow?

LAING: Oh, I think so, there can't be any doubt about that. It certainly sharpened my perception of knots and binds and all that sort of thing that I've since written quite a lot about. I think it was either that or going under the effects of that sort of thing which, if you can't see through, does seem to be the immediate factor that many people can't stand. Certainly my mother was a past master of that sort of tricky number.

CLARE: And then the choice of medicine, it was bound up with this question of suffering, the relief of suffering, understanding suffering, cracking the warps of brain and mind?

LAING: Well, I'd got myself into quite an intensely painful, spiritual, religious quandary over the issue of the existence of God which assumed almost life and death proportions. It still bothers me, things like that, the meaning of things. One thing about suffering was that I could not reconcile myself to the sort of God that I wanted to believe in, as a loving God who seemed to be responsible for a set-up in which so much pain was occurring. There was also the question what is death? Is there a life before death? What are we doing here? Where do we come from? Where are we going to? Who are we? Why are we? What are we? Some people say that we are not even alive now, that we are ghosts, that this is death and when we die we enter life and so forth and so on. And in the Calvinist world a great deal is placed on your salvation, on what you believe.

CLARE: What if I said to you that you were too sensitive to be a doctor?

LAING: I don't know whether it's a question of too sensitive. I haven't been able to do what a lot of doctors are able to do and many people, most people are able to do which is to keep their sensitivity within a fairly formally ordered frame of conduct. I get tossed and turned.

CLARE: One of the things I wondered was the extent to which that old adage applies, namely that senior physicians used to go on about not getting too close to the patient in general medicine, not getting too close to the patient in psychiatry indeed. The truth that was supposed to be at the heart of it was that if you did enter into what you've called 'The Golgotha of the spirit' it could destroy you, that you could be overwhelmed by that which you were there to try in some detached sense to cope with.

LAING: I've never been personally tempted to follow someone

over the edge, no. I don't like distracted and disordered and confused and bewildered states of mind, I do not like them at all. I'm very sorry for someone who's trapped in a state of mind like that, but I've got no desire to share it. You know the best way to get a drowning man, to rescue him, is not to fall into the river or the sea oneself but to stay in the lifeboat.

CLARE: Is this a change in you?

LAING: No.

CLARE: Well, I ask that because in the earlier days at times you used to suggest, partly in the poetic way in which you wrote, when you got to know what were called 'schizophrenics' – when you lived and talked and ate and drank and spoke and slept in their proximity and so on, you began to have actually grave doubts at distinguishing their experiences from your own.

LAING: This is very instructive because I realised that what you see is very largely conditioned by the way you look and it was actually possible to look at someone and see something else than that.

CLARE: But the difference you've just earlier identified that one is a distracted, tortured, agonised person?

LAING: Yes that's my view, that this is one man's view . . .

CLARE: That of a clinical psychiatrist who's seen many such people and been very close to a large number?

LAING: Sure. I don't think that someone who's in what a clinical psychiatrist would recognise as a psychotic state is any better or worse. I complained against the denigration of experience and the dehumanisation of the patient, but in doing so I wanted to bring them back into the ordinary human fold.

CLARE: Do you ever worry, do you worry particularly about your own sanity?

LAING: Um . . .

CLARE: Of losing it?

LAING: I've had spasms at times, fortunately never long-lasting fear in that respect. The thing that I think that has beset me most in my own personal life has really been depression. Two subjects I've never written about that I've been thinking that it might do me a lot of good just to write about are so-called heavy drinking, or alcoholism and depression. I'm quite a typical type of cryptopsychomotoretardation depressive – that is if you were to describe the sort of state that you get up in the morning, you're usually tireder than when you went to bed, it's a real drag, but you can push yourself through it. It's a driving, if you keep it up you're driving with the brakes on. It tends to get better somewhere in the middle of the day. The mood changes in the late afternoon and then most people who are in this sort of thing are taking tranquillisers or they've had to resort to alcohol. You mix it all and then by night time you're very tired and very wide awake. You can't get to sleep and then I know quite a number of people, as you must also, who take enormous numbers of sleeping tablets, plus half a bottle of brandy or something like that, to knock themselves over and then they wake up in the morning feeling worse than ever and so forth. Well that type of thing is the sort of thing that I've mainly been beset with in the last ten years of my life or so.

CLARE: Has that bleakness ever got so depressing that it wouldn't take much for you to end it all yourself?

LAING: Oh, yes, oh definitely. Fortunately never as part of this clinical picture, I've never actually entertained suicidal thoughts and I've always had a sort of fear of being ungrateful to the powers that be and so on for the life that I've had because, although I can get into miserable states of mind, it is always a tremendously consoling thought to look at other people who are infinitely worse off than oneself, if one's got the nerve to be consoled by that thought. I've got to live through this but I'm not going to buy it. About twenty years ago I was very frightened I was going to run into a real Scottish involutional melancholia.

CLARE: Let me ask you something. Supposing you were to become profoundly psychomotoretarded, profoundly depressed, suicidal, what would you want someone like me to do? If anything, indeed.

LAING: I would want whoever was taking my case over to make sure that I hadn't anything rational to worry about in terms of obligation, commitment, duties, etc. etc. that feed a sense of guilt and worthlessness and failure and then to transport my body to some nursing home and if you had any drugs that you thought would get me into a brighter state of mind and not be so completely given over to the effort to raise a finger or . . .

CLARE: Which is necessary in some severe depressions.

LAING: Yes I've felt that, I've felt like that, I've sometimes got terribly depressed.

CLARE: For long?

LAING: And for no known reason.

CLARE: Would it last long?

LAING: Well, in a sub-acute way I think I've been quite depressed, not all the time but in considerable patches for about the last ten years. I don't believe that the cause of worry is what one worries about because I know that I can look at exactly the same things when I'm not depressed and I see exactly the same things and they don't depress me. It's not so much things that depress me but it is completely senseless, and that's one of the depressive things about it – a completely senseless and inexplicable and opaque and infinitely boring state of sort of downness, flatness, lack of zest, lack of pleasure, lack of interests.

CLARE: I've asked lots of people this, not just in these kind of programmes but in my own clinic. What is it that sees us through? Family? Your wife?

LAING: That isn't one of the happy areas of my life at the moment, nor has it been for a number of years, neither for my wife nor for me and that's an occasion for sadness, but again not necessarily an occasion for depression, but not also a place of consolation.

CLARE: You've written in Volume One of your autobiography about a cycle that you half anticipate. You say 'Something overtook my father's father when he was in his fifties, and my father was a youth. Something overtook my father when he was in his fifties and I was a youth, I'm in my fifties and my son's a youth. I feel rocked by waves of hundreds of years.' What overtook your father? The only thing I could find out in that chain, what overtook your father when you were a youth and he was in his fifties was that he had something like a nervous breakdown. Is that what you're getting at?

LAING: Yes. For some reason my father's father, when my father was fourteen or fifteen, is said to have given up his career as a naval architect and a successful man about town and taken to whisky and sitting by the fire and doing nothing. My father was precipitated from school into a shipyard as an apprentice, a fact that he never forgave his father for, the necessity for him to break his education like that. I was a bit older, seventeen I think when my father had what would be called a nervous breakdown, certainly an anxiety neurosis with paranoid inflexion. He was in a state of trepidation, obsessed with the thought that his superior at work, who was about to retire, was going to try to do him in before he retired so that he wouldn't get promoted to that position. Well I was frightened in my forties, getting into my fifties, that I would run into some version of that cycle, sort of recycling itself down the generations that I've seen so often before, you know clinically in other people's family history, like sort of time bombs that await you in life. You think you've worked all through and you're out of it and then, specific to a certain age, you run into something that you never anticipated and there you go again and hopefully it's just a bad patch and you're out of it and you're never home and dry.

CLARE: What does the drinking do for you?

LAING: Well, it does different things. I started drinking as a student in Glasgow. When I go up to Glasgow people in some pubs don't even know that I don't live in Glasgow, I've never lost touch with the city, or with my sort of network of friends all of whom drink, all of whom drink by English standards, you know, an incredible amount. So I have become what we call a seasoned drinker. It's got all the different functions that drink can have, I'm in two minds about drinking just now. I've never felt that drinking has stopped me doing anything that I wanted to do. I don't feel that I'm impaired mentally, but I'm not sure that I'm prepared to accept a type of heavy drinking, ageing Scotsman as a sort of character type.

CLARE: Why would you quit? Why would you just write it out of the Laingian experience? Why would you just turn it off, why would you do that?

LAING: Why would I do it? I don't like not remembering what happened the morning after the night before. I used to not mind that.

CLARE: You've written somewhere, you said 'I saw love as crucified, but I could not see the resurrection,' then you said 'that was my nightmare, it is still.' Does this relate still to this search for meaning, for some kind of religious, with a small 'r' I suppose, explanation of what your life, what my life, what anybody's life is about?

LAING: Well, I think I've given up in one sense searching for a meaning. It's totally beyond my efforts. But the sense of futility and pointlessness is one of the themes of the depressive mood, you know the typical Scottish Calvinist involutional melancholic type of religious nihilistic ruminations. So I'm tarred with that brush, I haven't the faintest idea whether it's genetic but I think it's culture, very culture-bound.

CLARE: And when you look back at your life, can you counter these depressive ruminations with any sense of achievement?

LAING: Well the trouble is, as you know, it's very dangerous to try to think of anything comforting when you're depressed because of the skill with which one can undermine it – 'That's what I did in the past but what am I doing now, what's that got to do with me now?'

CLARE: We are sometimes seen by outsiders as a strange breed. Indeed it's said of psychiatrists that they are as mad as their patients. I don't know what the origin of these kinds of views of psychiatrists are because as you and I know they're a very wide and varied bunch. But is there some truth do you think at the heart of such a notion, to enter into a dialogue coming to terms with disturbance in oneself?

LAING: Undoubtedly there are some psychiatrists who have told me themselves and I've known over the years that because of the problematics of their own states of mind they've been attracted to this subject in particular and some I think have found it quite therapeutic as it were, professionally being paid to look into these issues which are both personal and of much wider relevance than just mere personal self-indulgence. That's quite a good contract.

CLARE: You don't describe yourself like that?

LAING: Oh I think the texture of the social and emotional life of my patients and what preoccupies them and what preoccupies me has a great deal in common, but I also recognise that a lot of people never very much think about the things that psychiatrists think about and so that when they hear psychiatrists talking shop they think that the psychiatrists are as crazy as their patients. I don't think that's true actually. I mean I've known a number of pretty eccentric psychiatrists but I've never known a psychiatrist who I would say was clinically psychotic or very far gone in some state of psychological ruination or confusion who was a practising psychiatrist.

CLARE: And in terms of your practice as a psychiatrist, does it have any bearing on the glooms, on the swings, the moods that you describe? Or are they unrelated?

LAING: I think the discipline of seeing patients, even when I'm feeling very down myself, is a real lifeline for me at times. It makes me address myself to someone else's problems and not get caught up in recycling my own to myself. I think that's one of the major issues clinically you might say about depression that you can either decide to keep going or that you're going to collapse and let yourself go. But then there's all the risk of incurring self-contempt for doing that when one's narcissism and pride is offended by the humiliating circumstances of admitting that one's at the end of one's ether and collapses. Well some people do that and make a mess of it. I would much rather consult someone like you before I got to that stage, but if I don't have to go as far as that, it is very salutary and refreshing to be able to address yourself to something else than that self-preoccupation of depression. A lot of people get very impatient with it who are not depressed themselves. You know there's a sort of terrible boring way that depressed people go on to you about nothing else but themselves. It's of no interest to anyone else and it's got no interest to them either, but if you get into that sort of thing it's very difficult to stop it.

CLARE: One of your reasons for entering medicine was that it might, in a sense, cast some light on the mystery of suffering. Now it didn't.

LAING: Not essentially, no.

CLARE: Is that because it couldn't, it was just the wrong question or that there's something missing at the heart of medicine?

LAING: No, I don't think so. I think it's really a theological question that one couldn't expect medicine to answer.

CLARE: No. What do you make of the fact that there are other people who have a theological answer, who have formulated what seems to them an explanation of life and death?

LAING: Well I can't say that I have. What do I think of people who have? Well at the very least good luck to them, and at the very most, if they have found a reconciliation for suffering, life, death and spiritual terms which is consistent and coherent and true, then I very much regret that such a vision hasn't come my way. I'm not unaware of the words that could be used to formulate such a view of things, but it hasn't come my way that I've been able to have that type of joyous clear shining eyes that some people who devote themselves to suffering have. If it's true I hope that I can see it's true, and if it's not true then I would rather be in a state of confusion than believe something that is consoling which isn't true. I don't want to trade in the truth for illusion.

Claire Rayner

In September 1988 I flew to Sacramento, courtesy of the BBC, to interview John Freeman. Freeman, now in his seventies and Visiting Professor of International Relations at the Unversity of California, had been one of the BBC's most accomplished stars in the early days of current affairs programmes such as *Panorama*, had edited the *New Statesman*, had been appointed High Commissioner to India and Ambassador to Washington by Harold Wilson and was chairman of London Weekend Television for thirteen years. But his name was remembered (and this, I found irritated him enormously) not so much for these achievements but for the fact that he had undertaken a series of some fifty television interviews during the late fifties and early sixties entitled *Face to Face*. The series was to become and remain a benchmark for in-depth and probing interviews on radio and television. My visit to Freeman was to record an interview which would be broadcast along with a selection of the most famous or infamous of the *Face to Face* interviews to mark the thirty years that had passed since they had first been broadcast.

The *Face to Face* interviews which most people recall were those Freeman conducted with Carl Jung, Evelyn Waugh, Tony Hancock and Gilbert Harding. Harding, one of the great broadcasting stars of the 1950s, and associated with such programmes as *The Brains Trust* and *Twenty Questions*, has been described by Paul Donovan in *The Radio Companion* as 'cantankerous, self-opinionated, extraordinarily rude, emotional and deeply insecure'. In September 1960 he was interviewed by John Freeman. Asked about his mother's death, Harding started to cry. It caused a sensation. While Freeman was heavily criticised at the time (and his cold, clipped, matter-of-fact interrogatory style as Harding wept didn't exactly encourage a feeling on the part of viewers that any genuine empathy was to be found in the studio), the event burned itself into the collective television unconscious. This was revelatory, psychological, clinical probing at its most effective and detached best.

In fact, as Freeman quickly made plain to me, far from being a carefully thought out, planned and executed revelation, it had all been a dreadful mistake. He, Freeman, had doubted that for all his talk Harding had ever encountered death and so asked him about it. To Freeman's horror, his subject revealed his mother had just died and then the pain of his attachment to her and his homosexual feelings uncontrollably gushed forth. Had he known would he have asked Harding the question? Certainly not was Freeman's crisp reply.

So when Claire Rayner, the agony aunt, broke down in tears during my interview with her in July 1988 comparisons, for the most part uninvited, were made with the Harding/Freeman episode. Inevitably, there was criticism. Why, when I realised from the outset that there were things about her childhood about which she preferred not to speak, that she preferred to leave at 'the bottom of my pond' and get on with living, why did I not leave it at that and move on to something else? Why, when she broke down and wept, did I not respect her suffering and change direction?

What those who ask such questions don't realise is that I knew that Claire Rayner knew that I would ask these questions. I knew she knew not merely because she had heard other interviews in the series. She knew because this was not the first time she had been interviewed by me. In 1982 I recorded a television series entitled *Motives* involving a number of subjects including Petula Clark, George Best and Richard Ingrams. The interview I did with Claire Rayner was for a variety of reasons, in the main technical, never shown. During it I sensed that behind her jolly bonhomie and breathless reassurance lay darkness and pain. On that occasion she used the image 'mud at the bottom of the pool' but kept me at bay and the interview ended without me being any the wiser as to what had happened. When, six years later, I invited her to sit in the Chair I believed that if she did not want to talk about what still distressed her she would turn down the invitation. The fact that she promptly accepted convinced me that she was prepared to talk. Indeed, I was moved to wonder whether she might actually want very much to talk about it.

She did break down uncontrollably, reduced to 'jelly' she was to say herself later, when I observed of her childhood memory, 'You mean time hasn't dulled it, or your method of coping with it hasn't defused it of its agony.' Some of her distress is heard in the programme but most of it was cut after Michael Ember, my producer, and I discussed it. We had no desire to broadcast such distress in its entirety. What remained was necessary to indicate something of the emotional intensity which mere reference to events now over forty years old still could cause. We were surprised by the impact of what remained. But I did feel and I still do that, given Claire Rayner's occupation, which is to purvey advice, reassurance, solace, sympathy and support to the thousands who seek it from her, it was important to discover whether she really was the composed, controlled superwoman she occasionally personified. Is the childhood mud related to the adult caring, I ask? I could have asked whether in examining and commenting on other people's miseries she repeatedly confronts and exorcises her own. I do make plain to her the fact that patients, clients, people who write to agony aunts often wonder just how healthy and mature and competent these appointed and self-appointed therapists and counsellors and agony aunts actually are.

I do suspect that Claire Rayner did want to talk with me about her background. Perhaps she wondered what those people who chose her (along with Felicity Kendal) as a 'role model' for women would make of the revelations that she had been rejected and abused as a child, that these experiences had marked her teenage and adult development and that to this day she still carried the scars. During the interview, she is unconvincingly dismissive of my suggestion that she worries that her image and role as an agony aunt might suffer. Her forceful tendency to equate talking about unhappy childhood experiences with a sort of self-indulgent stirring of a muddy pool is an attitude which is not uncommon amongst those who are to be found helping others to talk, self-analyse, reveal.

Wittingly or unwittingly, it contributes to the fantasy wherein there are healthy, integrated, mature people on the one hand and broken, impaired and disintegrated people on the other. Claire Rayner doesn't see much point in digging up the past 'if you can't do anything about it' which begs a question she doesn't beg with other people. They 'dig up the past' and present it to her and she, in her own intimitable way, tries to help them do something about it. Without meaning to, I felt she tended to imply, as tough, matter-of-fact, practical nurses often do, that getting about and energetically doing things is eminently superior to simply talking about them. But, and this lay at the heart of this interview, rushing about doing things can sometimes be a substitute for sitting down and taking a look at what is actually going on inside you, what distress or unhappiness is propelling you into action in the first place. In fact, the response to the programme, both from the critics and from the listening public, bore out my reassurance to her after the recording. The overwhelming judgement was that she appeared as a more rounded, more sympathetic, less bossy and authoritarian figure. The mystery is why anyone occupying the position she does could have believed otherwise. Of course there are those who want their doctors, advisers, therapists to be perfect, who project on to them fantasies of omnipotence to match their own nagging convictions of impotence and help-lessness. But most people in pain and trouble want those who help them to know what pain and trouble are about. They don't of course want their carers to be crippled by doubt or suffering or the scars of early deprivation but neither do they want them to be possessed of superhuman qualities, to be above the dissatisfaction and demoralisation of everyday life.

Claire Rayner is occasionally portrayed by her critics and cartoonists as a starchy, no-nonsense, over-bearingly gooey and motherly know-all inclined to reduce all human suffering, physical and psychological, to a box of tissues, an emotional band-aid and a dollop of good wholesome, homemade advice. It is her *Spitting Image* image. Whatever else about this inter-view, it provides little support for such a portrait. I do not believe it harmed her and neither do I think she thinks it did.

In all probability it did not do much one way or the other. It is after all just one more interview. But, if it did have an effect, I hope and trust it was the effect that starting out on this series back in 1982 I hoped might occasionally be produced, namely the reminder that even the most successful, competent, efficient are not without their muddy pools – but they have managed to arrive at ways of limiting the damage. I have been intrigued and somewhat amused to discover from reading Paul Donovan's *The Radio Companion* that largely as a result of the *In the Psychiatrist's Chair* interview, Claire Rayner decided to host a BBC Radio 2 series entitled *Myself When Young* in which various people are encouraged to talk in a light, enjoyable reminiscing fashion about their formative years. Ebullient to the last, she insists on the value of emphasising the positive, identifying the shimmering fish, the vigorous plants, the nourishing oxygen in that childhood pool leaving me and those like me to poke around in the mud, the weeds and the decay. Horses for courses as she puts it and who am I to argue with her?

CLARE: Claire Berenice Rayner was born on January 22nd 1931. Both her parents were Jewish and she was the eldest of four children. Her brother is a producer, director and screenwriter in Hollywood. Her two sisters live in Canada. Aged eight, at the outbreak of war, she was evacuated and when the war ended she attended The City of London School for Girls before training to be a nurse at The Royal Northern Hospital. However she always wanted to become a doctor and did start working to obtain the necessary qualifications for medical school, but marriage intervened. She married her husband Desmond in 1957. They have two sons and one daughter. Following the birth of her first child she began to write, first for nursing magazines, then a book on the maternity services, then novels. Now she is the best known TV and broadcasting agony aunt in the country, has written over seventy books, and her multi-faceted business is managed by her husband. Claire Rayner, how do you feel about talking about yourself?

RAYNER: Not terribly comfortable, I don't think it's what I'm for, I'm for trying to be useful to other people mostly and I'm for telling stories and so on. So you might ask why the hell I'm here, since if I don't like it, why did I agree. I've been asking myself you know all the way here.

CLARE: You don't like talking about yourself.

RAYNER: Not in depth, no.

CLARE: Why?

RAYNER: I daresay there's a lot of mud in there. I think, I decided this a long time ago, that there's a lot of mud at the bottom of my pond.

CLARE: You know that?

RAYNER: I know that, yes, I'm not a fool. I know perfectly well there are all sorts of muddy things in my past history that are potentially damaging. But there's a lot of mud there and on top of that there's about three inches of clear water.

CLARE: When you say potentially damaging, you mean they haven't damaged you yet?

RAYNER: Not to my knowledge. Look, a long time ago I came to the conclusion that the real skill in life was to make your neuroses work for you rather than against you.

CLARE: When did you discover that?

RAYNER: Oh, heavens, I don't know, nursing sometime. I couldn't say exactly when, but it was a long time ago.

CLARE: Well, put it this way, when were you nothing like as ebullient and together as you appear now?

RAYNER: Ah, 'appear', bless you for that. Ebullient I've always been, you know the Andrews Liver Salts type.

CLARE: You said, 'It wasn't what I'm for,' namely looking into yourself; you're engaged in helping other people.

RAYNER: I'm still nursing, that's what I was trained for.

CLARE: Yes, but immediately people will wonder, as they do about my profession and any of the caring professions, whether there is a connection between the mud and the caring?

RAYNER: Yes, absolutely. The thing that started me off as a writer, perhaps, was a memory I have of being sent for by my sister tutor, during my second year and she said 'Nurse

Chetwynd, the BMA, the British Medical Association, are having an essay competition for nurses and you will enter,' and in those days you did pull your forelock and say, 'Yes, Sister.' I'd never dreamed of writing, but she saw something I didn't. So I entered it and the subject was, I remember, 'Is Nursing a vocation?' To write the piece I went round talking to all the people I trained with to find out why they were nursing and I found out, to my great comfort at the time, that every one of them was in nursing for some sort of ulterior motive. They all had a need that was being satisfied by the work they were doing. So I felt better, 'cos I knew I had needs that were being satisfied.

CLARE: What were they?

RAYNER: I wanted security without too much emotional involvement, and I discovered fairly early on that the sensible thing to do with past pain and past distress of your own is to use the alchemist's stone on it. You can turn it into something useful instead of sitting there, moaning over your past and saying, 'Oh, God, I suffered.' What's the point of that?

CLARE: But I'm still a little puzzled by the fact that very quickly you said 'mud at the bottom of the pool', and briskly talked about getting on and contrasting that with sitting and being miserable. I'm unclear the extent to which you have actively confronted it, that you would talk about it. In most of the things written about you there is nothing. There is just the bald statement. You were an evacuee, but not just that, you were a Jewish family in the East End, but I sense nothing of the warmth. Your father is poorly described, likewise your mother, your sisters are in Canada, your brother is in Hollywood, but even long before that, I sense nothing, I feel nothing about what went on then.

RAYNER: That box is closed because . . .

CLARE: Well, was it ever opened?

RAYNER: Oh, I've opened it personally, quietly to myself.

CLARE: To anyone else? To an agony aunt?

RAYNER: Why, what's the point?

CLARE: Others do it.

RAYNER: No, well I don't want to. I'd rather take the contents of that box, let it be mud at the bottom of the pond as I say, and support a couple of healthy growths. And the growths it supports is the work I do as an agony aunt, as a medical journalist and so forth, a teacher if you like, I'm still nursing.

CLARE: Isn't it an irony that so many other people are doing quite the opposite with you. Not only are they confronting it, they're actually doing it often in public newspapers, on radio, even on television?

RAYNER: I know. That's their need, and it's horses for courses. If that's what they need, fine, I'm not too happy to help in that direction. My needs are different. The way I handle my problems, my past and all of that, is I filter a lot of it into fiction, a lot of it's in my novels in its own way, and I use it in that way.

CLARE: But I sense a panic in you that it might be looked at?

RAYNER: I don't want it to be, why should I?

CLARE: But here you are.

RAYNER: Maybe it's the fun of fencing with you, Anthony, I don't know, but I don't see any point in, in digging up past misery if you can't do anything about it.

CLARE: Would it be past miseries?

RAYNER: Oh, I think so, yes.

CLARE: It would be painful?

RAYNER: Yes, so I don't want to.

CLARE: Why do you think people do it?

RAYNER: Because they haven't resolved how to handle it themselves. I've found a way to handle past pain.

CLARE: How?

RAYNER: I work. It's the work I do.

CLARE: You mean you forget it.

RAYNER: I perhaps forget it, and perhaps turn it into something useful and perhaps turn it into, as I say, the lead of the distress into, I hope, the gold of a story.

CLARE: Does it work?

RAYNER: Well, I'm doing fine most of the time, most of the time.

CLARE: I've read what you write, you reflect on the extent to which we are what made us. In the lost boyhood of Judas,

Christ was betrayed – the notion that we are formed by the past. Let's take a situation with which you're very commonly involved because it is written to you many times. When you come to a life-stage where you are forced to look again at what made you, like marriage, where you become the wife your mother was, where you become the mother your mother was?

RAYNER: Well, I'd made a deliberate conscious attempt to make sure I wasn't what they had been.

CLARE: Well, what was your mother?

RAYNER: Not an easy person to live with, highly manipulative. She was very controlling, a child. What's that lovely thing I read in a French joke book? I feel like *un petit, d'un petit,* a child of a child, not a very adequate person, both too young and, and unprepared, all that; but you know, as I say I don't really want to go on and on about it, because I don't see any point.

CLARE: But you never go on and on about it.

RAYNER: No, no, I don't want to.

CLARE: No, my point is that in any other individual, I think a bricklayer or a cricketer or even perhaps a judge, I might leave it, because I'm tempted to believe that those particular preoccupations and many others aren't necessarily involved with what makes us tick. But in your case I think I am justified in pushing a little, because you're a woman who gives freely of advice to people on how to live and how to cope with savagery and set-back and brutality, child abuse and so on.

RAYNER: I hope I'm not the end of anyone's road. But this is a very valid point.

CLARE: Hence people are interested to know how have you done it?

RAYNER: Yes.

CLARE: And here you're telling me you've done it by actually ignoring it.

RAYNER: By taking a deep breath and getting up and standing there and saying, 'Am I going to spend any more time looking back over my shoulder at things that can't be changed, or am I going to get on with living.' And I made that latter choice.

CLARE: When did you do this looking back?

RAYNER: Oh, at various stages, Anthony; I mean I'm fifty.

CLARE: But when? I mean isn't it true, Claire, you actually haven't looked at it much.

RAYNER: No, I absolutely agree. I don't see any point, and interestingly enough my brother does, too. We, we don't see a great deal of each other, because he's in Hollywood and I'm here, but I did actually see him earlier this year. We talked a bit about this and we both agreed, he's a very successful writer, we both agreed that it was horrible while it lasted, but it's been bloody useful ever since.

CLARE: All right, well then, let's take you drawing on it. In this same series I talked to Anthony Burgess. There's a man who draws and writes on it. You can see hidden, shadowy, but nonetheless perceptible, reflections of what he's been through in his extraordinary background. Now, presumably you're saying you do something similar. Now, when you're doing it, are you saying that the spectre of the past is there beside you as you write about, I don't know, somebody's childhood, somebody's marriage, somebody's experience?

RAYNER: Sometimes. Not marriage, because my own is very, very comfortable. Oh, I can remember, yes, and I will to an extent draw on that. I mean, I know what it's like to be a beaten child.

CLARE: Leaving aside the question of what's the point, put that aside for a second, the point of looking at it. Let's put aside the point. Would it be painful? I mean acutely painful? You're not sure?

RAYNER: Almost certainly, yes, almost certainly it would.

CLARE: You mean time hasn't dulled it, or your method of coping with it hasn't defused it of its agony?

RAYNER: No.

CLARE: It was that bad.

RAYNER: Mmmn.

CLARE: Let me ask you something else. In what way do you think it has shaped you?

RAYNER: I think it has made me reasonably resilient, believe it or not. I do bounce back, which is quite useful.

CLARE: Let me press you about my own process. Do you think that psychiatry at times overdoes the preoccupation with the past?

RAYNER: For some people it might. I think for some people it might be like playing that gramophone record over and over and over again, and sooner or later, for God's sake, you've got to stop rehearsing it.

CLARE: But you've never done that?

RAYNER: I know, but . . .

CLARE: You keep using this image of over and over again but you've never done it once!

RAYNER: Not in public, no, this was what you were talking about.

CLARE: Or with someone?

RAYNER: No, not with anyone else.

CLARE: Desmond, your husband?

RAYNER: A little, a little. Some of it, but why inflict it on him?

CLARE: You feel that's what it would be doing? You don't see it as a sharing?

RAYNER: No. He had his own problems.

CLARE: You're quite right to say why should I share it with you, but let's leave that for a second. Don't you see that as long as you are what you are outwardly no one really knows you?

RAYNER: Well, that's fine. What does it matter? I don't necessarily want everyone to know me.

CLARE: I didn't say everyone, I said no one. You do that all the time.

RAYNER: I think Des does, I think Des does, yes.

CLARE: How? Intuitively?

RAYNER: Partly that and, damn it, we've been married thirty-one years.

CLARE: But there are things you haven't talked about.

RAYNER: Oh, very little, very little . . .

CLARE: Let me ask you something else. Why have you got this image of 'over and over'?

RAYNER: I do know people who are trapped, and I've come across them in letters and so on, who are trapped in an eternal rehashing of past pains.

CLARE: Is that what you're frightened of, you might do that?

RAYNER: I think so, I don't think I want to do that.

CLARE: You fear that once you did it you'd go on doing it?

RAYNER: You've got to step off the roundabout and start to live. Get up, brush yourself down and get on with it. It's the best thing I ever did. You see there was a time when I did just flounder from situation to situation, not really thinking about where I was going, what I was doing. I was just, just living day by day and getting nowhere. And I think I came back to England from Canada, where it had all been all rather awful, and actually had to look at who I was and what I was and what I was going to do. Was I going to go on being the person I'd been, you know this sort of nineteen-year-old mess as it were, or start, use it as a fresh start, coming back home, back to London?

CLARE: Were you a nineteen-year-old mess?

RAYNER: Oh, I think so, yes, I'd been in hospital a long time. I'd had a long period of illness, you know psychiatric illness and I wanted no more of it. The interesting thing was I developed thyrotoxicosis when I came back to England, having been in hosiptal for quite some time in Canada. Well, I'd been dumped, frankly.

CLARE: How do you mean you'd been dumped?

RAYNER: I'd been dumped in hospital, I mean literally dumped by my parents. I was sixteen and it was between sixteen and nineteen.

CLARE: They were there, you were there.

RAYNER: They were there and I was there because they persuaded me to join them which I didn't want to do. But because I was under twenty-one they were financially responsible for me and because they were financially feckless they didn't want to know. I did become ill, you know, I was a sort of stormy adolescent, and having all sorts of problems.

CLARE: And they put you in a hospital, a psychiatric hospital?

RAYNER: Yes, and dumped me.

CLARE: For how long?

RAYNER: Oh, about fifteen, sixteen months.

CLARE: And what has that left you with?

RAYNER: A great deal of concern for the welfare of people who aren't well. Quite a fighter on their behalf. In case you hadn't noticed.

CLARE: Were you very anxious, were you an anxious girl?

RAYNER: Well, I suppose so.

CLARE: I mean who loved you then?

RAYNER: I think I thought of myself as the Vicar of Bray, remember the song 'The Vicar of Bray'?

CLARE: You mattered to no one.

RAYNER: 'I care for nobody, no, not I and nobody cares for me.' It had a lot going for it, emotional freedom. Really I mean not having to worry about someone else's feelings or needs, you know.

CLARE: Did you ever have any contact with psychiatry since then?

RAYNER: No way, not on your nelly. Apart from you.

CLARE: In that sense, what do you think people would make of it?

RAYNER: I don't really care.

CLARE: But that isn't the reason you haven't talked about it?

RAYNER: No, it's nothing to do with that. No, it's not relevant anymore. It's over.

CLARE: Did this image which we'll stick with, the mud at the bottom of the pond, did it affect you when you were getting married or when you were involved with Desmond?

RAYNER: I didn't want to get married.

CLARE: You didn't want to?

RAYNER: I wanted to live with him but Des was much more determined. He said if we don't get married we won't last and he was determined, he needed security.

CLARE: And you didn't want to get married because?

RAYNER: No, but I wanted him. Because my only example of marriage had been awful, I mean the one I'd grown up in, as it were. And for the same reason I didn't want children. I didn't want to inflict the same things on them, or didn't want the risk of doing it. In the event it's worked exceedingly well and I'm very grateful to them.

CLARE: Now what is the reason I ask you some of this, what is the justification? Let me give you just a small example, I'd be interested to hear your view on this. It is said of many doctors, many nurses, that they have actually a lower threshold for pain than their patients, that they kind of rush in because they cannot bear it. Would you see yourself like that? Very sensitive to pain?

RAYNER: Not my own and not physical pain.

CLARE: What about watching television?

RAYNER: Oh, it depends on what it is. I get very distressed, yes.

CLARE: Stories like child abuse, violence, what do you do?

RAYNER: Work a bit harder.

CLARE: Do you watch it?

RAYNER: Oh, yes, you can't hide. I try to find some use in it, something I can do that will be useful. The thing that's depressing about pain and trouble and disaster is helplessness. I mean helplessness makes you depressed or maybe depression and helplessness is the same disease.

CLARE: Which is what you remember?

RAYNER: Yes, perhaps I do . . . but helplessness, powerlessness . . .

CLARE: Why didn't you stay in nursing?

RAYNER: I got pregnant and in 1960 there was no way they'd let me.

CLARE: You were never tempted to go back? But you would have been a damn good nurse.

RAYNER: Oh, dear, I was, okay, I'm going to stick my neck out, I was, I know I was, I did awfully well.

CLARE: Would you have been, you know, the damn good ward sister who knew more than the young doctors who ran the ward?

RAYNER: I was by the time I finished. I knew what I was doing, and I was fierce in protection of my patients, always, very fierce.

CLARE: How did you cope with patients dying, patients for whom you could do nothing, patients in pain?

RAYNER: It was awful, and when children were involved that was dreadful. I nearly quit at one point because it got so bad and I had a sister tutor, she's now very old and lives in Cornwall, and she was wonderful. I came off duty one night and went over to the nursing school, it was my second year, and I said 'Sister Bishop, I'm giving up, I can't stand it. It's been the most awful night. I feel like the little boy with his thumb in the dyke and I can't handle it and I'm going to give up.' And she said, 'Nurse Chetwynd, who do you think you are? God?' She said, 'Now you do what you can and you leave the rest to others. Now go to bed, get a day's sleep and come on duty tonight. I want no more of this nonsense.' And I said, 'Yes, Sister.' And she was right.

CLARE: Did you find religion useful?

RAYNER: Never, no, no, no, no. I would have liked to be religious and it must be very very comforting.

CLARE: Do you feel Jewish?

RAYNER: No, not particularly I'm afraid.

CLARE: Where was the extended Jewish family? That's the vision we have of the Jewish family in the East End.

RAYNER: Yes, yes, but it wasn't like that. Because when the war started in thirty-nine I was eight, we were scattered. We were flung apart as a family. We've never really made it back together again. There were, at that time on the periphery, a super grandmother and a marvellous aunt and other aunts and uncles, cousins, on my father's side. And I'm now very close to my paternal uncle and aunt whom I adore. They're wonderful people who also let me get on with the present you see, sensible.

CLARE: Do you have any prejudices?

RAYNER: Oh, masses of prejudices, of course I do.

CLARE: As a result of a certain kind of experience, for example, would you feel sometimes very cynical about the picture that's painted of warm, East End Jewish families?

RAYNER: Oh, very, yes, I'm very cynical about that.

CLARE: Are you a cynical person?

RAYNER: No, but I'm cynical about that, because I've been there.

CLARE: The romanticisation of the past?

RAYNER: Yes. I don't like the romanticisation of that. Some people get most cross with me when I write articles reminding people that the good old days weren't that good, that the past was as imbued with violence and abused children and cruelty, in many ways more so than the present. But people want to remember a golden past.

CLARE: Was there violence in your family?

RAYNER: Some, yes, yes.

CLARE: There was drinking?

RAYNER: No, never. Isn't that interesting? No, alcohol was not part of it.

CLARE: It didn't sour you about human nature?

RAYNER: Oh, no, not sour. I just think people can do better.

CLARE: Where did you get that from? Where was that model derived from? What about your evacuee families?

RAYNER: No that wasn't much fun. I kept running away, I hated it. Let's be honest. Not all the people who took East End evacuees were frightfully keen on the idea. There were some who took us for the seven and six a week I think it was the government gave. I have memories of finishing up with hands swollen and purple because of washing eggs, umpteen eggs. I'd been billeted on a chicken farm in Devonshire and remember washing eggs before going to school, hundreds and hundreds of these goddamn eggs. I can still remember doing it in ice cold water, because, you know, we were cheap labour for some people. Perhaps I was unlucky with some of the people I was billeted on. I can remember one family who were absolutely lovely in Yorkshire, in Keighley. By this time I was going to school. They were a lovely family called Exley who, who were unconditional, they gave unconditional acceptance. But a lot of the people, as I recall, that I was billeted on gave anything but unconditional acceptance. You had to be grateful and polite and do as you were told and keep out of sight and, and there was a lot of taunting – you know, 'we're fighting the war for the likes of you,' that sort of thing.

CLARE: Anti-semitism?

RAYNER: Oh, yes, then. so a lot of the running away, I think, was running away from, rather than back to, you know.

CLARE: What's your first really sustained, positive memory?

RAYNER: First memory?

CLARE: A sustained positive memory?

RAYNER: It didn't get good until I grew up, and then it got good.

CLARE: By grow up, you mean what age?

RAYNER: Well, when I came back to England, you know at about twenty, from then on it got good and it's been good ever since, and getting better and got better. I can tell you there are some strands – public libraries, public libraries from the time I was very young – now, they I remember with enormous gratitude.

CLARE: When you went to nursing, you actually went to City of London School for Girls. Was that a scholarship?

RAYNER: I got a scholarship, but that was by accident again. You see, I didn't know until I was quite old that I'm quite bright. In fact I am, you know, and I got the scholarship by an oversight, I swear to you, because at school I never did anything. School was one of the areas where I could actually impose my own will. I got this scholarship and it was a chance to go away to a school, although I only had a year or so there. There are great gaps, enormous gaps that are totally lost, which I rather resent in some ways. One of my sisters has remarkable recall, and she will tell me of things about my own past, and I say, 'Good heavens, did that happen?' and she says 'yes, surely you remember that?' and I say, 'No, it's all gone.'

CLARE: Do you believe in the notion of catharsis?

RAYNER: For some people, yes.

CLARE: But not for you?

RAYNER: I haven't risked it, as I say, all my neuroses are working in my favour at the moment, aren't they? Or seem to be. I think so mostly, I think so mostly. I enjoy my work. I've got a successful marriage as far as I can tell, to the best of my knowledge, three rather nice young adults that I can look at and say, 'Yes, they're all right,' and I don't think that's bad going.

CLARE: Your husband's very important?

RAYNER: Oh, yes, the sun rises and sets in him.

CLARE: As a support?

RAYNER: Yes. I think we're a bit of a joke in some sense. I mean we've been written about enough together, haven't we? And we've been portrayed by people – there have been snide cracks, you know, 'No one could be that content with each other,' but we are. We might be a little too dependent on each other which is not healthy. We both know it because it isn't terribly good to be totally dependent for your security on one other person, is it?

CLARE: Is your husband someone who belongs to the other category – who will let it all out?

RAYNER: No, no, he's the same as me. We talk to each other. Yes, he'll tell me things, yes. And yet, let me be fair, when he's hit a bad patch he's been willing to go into therapy which I wouldn't do.

CLARE: Have you hit a bad patch?

RAYNER: Oh, of course. Any number of them.

CLARE: What do you do?

RAYNER: I write another book or something and find another way of dealing with it.

CLARE: You mean writing is therapy?

RAYNER: It's the greatest therapy there is. It keeps all sorts of things at bay, doesn't it?

CLARE: But you've also written about the fact that the British aren't very good at grieving and that there's an awful lot of stiff upper lip and get on with living.

RAYNER: Yes, I haven't said they're not good at grieving so much as they're not good at public acceptance of grief, of others' grief. Now that's a different thing. Some people are better at grieving than others.

CLARE: But the reason we're not very good at it is that we basically think it's something that we shouldn't be doing.

RAYNER: Yes, I suppose so. I mean you won't see in Britain what you will see in some Mediterranean countries in particular, people keening and wailing and rolling together in their distress.

CLARE: Or even weeping.

RAYNER: Or even weeping in public. It's not considered good form at all, is it, in this country?

CLARE: What do you think?

RAYNER: I hate it if I do it myself, as you know. I mean I do get very bothered.

CLARE: Now?

RAYNER: Well, I hate it, yes. For me being in control of myself is important, probably over-controlled.

CLARE: Why did you say that?

RAYNER: That I'm over-controlled? Because I know it to be so. I suppose it's probably a good thing to let go sometimes.

CLARE: Is it because you think if you let go you wouldn't be able to stop letting go?

RAYNER: That's a possibility.

CLARE: Let me put to you that one of the reasons I started doing this series, the very first series, was I had a patient who knew I met people like you and wondered whether, behind all their apparent control, success and so on, they were people like her.

RAYNER: Of course we all are, everyone is.

CLARE: Yes, but you say that. They've only got it as an act of faith unless you, people like you, actually say that that's what they're like.

RAYNER: I don't know. It bothers me to display too much. Aren't I entitled to some bits to keep to myself?

CLARE: You're entitled to keep anything to yourself. This is in the nature of a discussion about why people reveal as much as they reveal. I mean you wouldn't by any means be the first or the last person in this series to talk about, for example, having had psychiatric treatment or been in hospital or been put there by somebody else, or been deprived of parental love, or anything. You wouldn't be the first and you won't be the last. What makes it of interest in relation to you much more so than in relation, as I say, to somebody not working in the field in which you work, is that it is crucially involved, surely, with what you are doing?

RAYNER: Yes, that's valid, that's fair. That's what drove me into nursing.

CLARE: Because nursing is staunching the blood.

RAYNER: Yes, I was trained, I was given a tool.

CLARE: And doesn't stir up the mud really.

RAYNER: No, it was a tool. It was a marvellous, useful tool.

CLARE: To do something.

RAYNER: To do something, to do something, to be useful, and, to the best of my knowledge, to do no harm.

CLARE: That's enormously rich and positive and isn't in any sense invalidated by you describing what made Claire Rayner Claire Rayner. How is that invalidated? What worries you?

RAYNER: I suppose it's the intrusion.

CLARE: The possibility that the edifice is shaken?

RAYNER: No, I don't think so.

CLARE: That people won't see you quite the same way?

RAYNER: No, I don't care about that particularly. I suppose it goes back to the training that the patient came first and it was their needs that were paramount and if you had needs of your own, hard luck.

CLARE: It's not that people's image of you would be shaken?

RAYNER: I think perhaps some of the usefulness would go, perhaps that's what it is. Perhaps some of the usefulness would go. Let me say I was sailing in a boat on difficult waters, would I feel right if I knew that the boat had once been badly damaged and had been carefully caulked? Would I not feel less safe, that's what it is?

CLARE: But you're not a cracked vessel.

RAYNER: Not any more I hope, no, I'm not any more, no.

CLARE: Those people who would be shaken by this revelation, that suggests to me that actually they've got a child's relationship with you, they see you as parental.

RAYNER: Yes, now that perhaps, yes, though that would be a pity, wouldn't it, because quite often one of the things you have to do with a job like mine is somehow slowly wean away the dependent one, because it's not good. The ones who want to go on writing letters and who want to just go on relating to what looks to them like a, quote – 'glamorous image' – unquote, and I have to sort of say, now you know that's not on and it's not quite like that. Did you know people could develop a transference by way of a letter? They can. It happens. One must be very kind, you've got to lead them away from it.

CLARE: Is it possible you wanted to change that?

RAYNER: What? That, that I don't want people to become dependent, you mean?

CLARE: Well, that you don't really want them to see you the way you're not.

RAYNER: I suppose, I just feel that it's private, it's personal. Do I have to 'strip my sleeve and show my scars and say these wounds got I on Crispin's Day?' Why?

CLARE: All right, but let's not go over the top. You've revealed certain things have happened. I haven't gone into the full details.

RAYNER: You better not!

CLARE: But I haven't. The point I'm making is that isn't it interesting the extent to which you use the extreme to prevent us looking at the middle? That's to say you say, 'going on and on', meaning 'I'd rather not talk this once about it.' You say, 'letting it all hang out and being frightfully personal', when in fact you've revealed just one or two very important things. Not for a minute do I demean them, because otherwise I wouldn't be doing this, nor do I think in any sense they demean you.

RAYNER: Well, that's a comfort perhaps, I don't know.

CLARE: But is that something you fear?

RAYNER: Perhaps so, perhaps.

CLARE: If you were to describe how you come across?

RAYNER: I have a pretty negative image of myself as I come across, noisy, pushy, arrogant perhaps, in fact bloody opinionated.

CLARE: Pollyannaish?

RAYNER: Oh, no, heaven! But there is an element in Pollyannaism that is not to be totally diminished and knocked. There was a long fashion for saying, 'Oh, God, how awful to play the glad game.' I hope everyone's read *Pollyanna* who's listening to this. Shall we remind them? Well, the 'glad game' was whatever happened to Pollyanna, this repellent American child, she found something good to say about it. So that when she was given a pair of crutches for a Christmas present, she was able to say, 'Well, I'm glad I don't need them,' I mean it's enough to set your teeth on edge. And at it's worst that's Pollyannaism. I mean it's sort of mawkish, sentimental gunge. But there are good things about Pollyannaism. The good thing is saying, 'Well, yes, that's pretty rotten but I could cope; I'll get up and dust myself off, get on with the next thing. Or, Yes that was horrid, but I'll use it, I'll put it in a book,' or, 'Well, there's always tomorrow.'

CLARE: Do you ever wish, irrationally no doubt, that you could confront your parents and get them to explain why it was all so dreadful.

RAYNER: Oh, but I know why.

CLARE: Why?

RAYNER: They were young and they were inadequate. There was a depression, they were poor, there were a whole lot of things.

CLARE: So it doesn't mystify you.

RAYNER: Oh, there's no mystery about it, there's no mystery.

CLARE: The lovelessness.

RAYNER: No, no mystery at all. I actually am beginning to be able to feel sorry for them, which is quite an achievement, isn't it really, when you think about it?

CLARE: Why, what did you feel for them?

RAYNER: Oh, it was fury and hate for a long time, but that's gone, mostly.

CLARE: Why are you now feeling sorry for them? What do you now know you didn't know then?

RAYNER: Well, they were so young, you see, and I can see what it does to people, and poverty of course. Their poverty was due to fecklessness as much as anything. Their family helped, my father's family helped them out over and over again. To this day people I meet, elderly people, who say,

'Oh, I could tell you stories about your father,' and I'd say, 'I know, I've heard, I've heard them.' He had enormous charm.

CLARE: Did he pretend to be what he was not?

RAYNER: Often, often.

CLARE: Did anyone know?

RAYNER: He was a great fantasiser.

CLARE: In detail, did anyone know him?

RAYNER: I wonder, I doubt it, I doubt it, poor man.

CLARE: And your mother, was she a pretty woman?

RAYNER: Oh, yes, very, and that of course was a terrible handicap, it is you know, prettiness. Yes, she was very pretty. You come to use it, you come to count on it too much, don't you think so? I mean I think the pretty woman has a lovely time to start with, but if she is allowed to use it and rely on it, it does let you down, mere prettiness. I've always been very grateful that that wasn't me, very grateful. A beauty I never was, thank God.

CLARE: The society in which we live is a very public society. Recently I read somewhere that you were amongst the most publicised or popular figures in Britain.

RAYNER: Somebody did a survey about what women want and they wanted to know how to sell things better to women, and they wanted to know who their role models were and to my absolute amazement I came second on the list, and I thought, 'Ye gods, that's an awful, awful responsibility.'

CLARE: Why, what's the responsibility?

RAYNER: What, to be a role model for other people? To say, 'Be like me and everything will be lovely'? That's a load of old codswallop. It isn't, you've got to be yourself. What was interesting, I found interesting, was at the top of the list was the actress Felicity Kendall and I thought that says it all, really, because they were only going for public images. In Felicity's case, as she herself said, she'd like to be the person they thought she was, the character she plays, and I suppose a bit of me would like to be the person that a lot of people clearly think I am, and that worried me too, because I'm not.

CLARE: You mean you'd like to be your own role model?

RAYNER: In a sense.

CLARE: What about the responsibility for them to know the real role model that you are, is there not a responsibility?

RAYNER: Yes, there is one I suppose. So maybe sitting here and saying this to Radio Four's audience will, will diminish some of it. You know people will say, 'Oh, well, that's not the role model I want. Good, I'll find another one.' Maybe that would be a good thing.

CLARE: Could you cope with that?

RAYNER: Yes, I think so, I hope so, gosh I hope so. I mean I don't necessarily want to be loved by the whole world, but I suspect I want to be loved by quite a chunk of it.

CLARE: Supposing they know a good deal more, for example that your background is much more traumatic, that you've come from a very different background from the way it now looks? What do you think that would do to your status as a role model?

RAYNER: Do you know, I don't know, I don't worry about it. It's just that, as I say, it is like taking your clothes off in public and at root you know I'm frightfully British at heart. There are things you don't do in public and I'm not sure, as I say, that showing your scars is a decent thing to do entirely, is it?

Sir James Savile

The interview with Jimmy Savile was not one of the easiest. Throughout he appeared exceedingly wary, edgy, like a prize-fighter on his toes, anticipating a flurry of hooks to the head, feinting, jabbing a little, constantly on the watch for a blow below the belt. He came dressed as usual in a tracksuit. He alternatively smoked and sucked on a cigar. He talked what is now his characteristic and distinctive brand of quick-fire, sixties patter. Within about ten minutes of the interview I knew what my problem was, whatever about his! Sir James Savile is a quintessentially self-made man, indeed he is *the* self-made man – and he is constantly, shrewdly, reshaping his creation to meet whatever are the needs of the immediate moment. His most brilliant discovery, during his early twenties, was that his flair for finding what people wanted and providing it would make his fortune. He now possesses an outstanding ability to play an astonishing range of roles – entrepreneur, disc-jockey, eccentric, devoted son, millionaire, prison warder, hospital porter, friend of the famous, confidant of royalty, knight of the realm, fool, jester, sage and pirate.

Rereading the interview, and indeed listening to the tape, I am struck by two recurrent themes – an emphasis on money and a denial of feelings. Going back through the press cuttings these preoccupations appear there too. Much is written of Savile's own wealth and the wealth he has made for others. Much is made too of his lack of emotional baggage in his life journey. There just does not seem to be anybody who can say or does say that he or she knows this man intimately.

In the interview, the issue of money arises almost irrespective of the questions asked. When I ask about his father, he is described as 'marvellous' and then the regret is quickly added that he didn't live 'to see a few of my quid'. When I ask about his mother, he replies, 'Perfectly ordinary. She had no money. She had another six to go at and my Dad.' When I inquire about his childhood he insists it was happy but money was scarce, then adds, 'I keep harping on about no money but if there's no money there's no money.' The memory he recalls from adolescence is pulling a picture of a Rolls Royce out of a book and pinning it up beside his wardrobe. Others, I might have observed but didn't, were pinning up pictures of Betty Grable and Dorothy Lamour. He tells me of his purchasing seventeen new Rolls Royces and when asked why, observes, 'I can go skint in a day.' He is determined to stay single and when asked what are the features that make him ideally suited to being a single man, he promptly answers that he has the ultimate luxury, 'I've got all the money that was ever printed.'

Throughout the interview, Jimmy Savile insists that he is a man without feelings. Perhaps he is. It is only in the cracks and crevices of the conversation that doubts lurk. Much, for example, is made of 'The Duchess' but much does not appear to amount to much. There are hints that being the 'not again' pregnancy, the seventh of seven in a household that was 'skint', may have left the young Jimmy not merely materially deprived but emotionally deprived too. The insistence on emotional independence, on travelling light and often, on keeping free of personal entanglements together with his obvious ability to adhere to such an emotionally spartan regimen do suggest someone with powerful reasons to shun intimacy. The one moment of poignancy concerns his mother's death. He spent five days with her, between her death and her funeral. Why? 'Once upon a time I had to share her with a lot of people . . . but when she was dead she was all mine.'

The newspapers at the time were intrigued. Some psychologically minded commentators speculated darkly on a seemingly morbid preoccupation with death, it having been widely reported earlier that he was rather drawn to the mortuary at St James's Hospital in Leeds (where he works occasionally as a porter), and this, together with the five days with the dead 'Duchess', seemed to suggest an unwholesome death complex. Perhaps he has one. People with a distaste for emotions, who place great value on predictability and control, who see life as incorrigibly messy and death as a frozen model of perfection, are half in love with death. The dead don't let you down, don't make demands, don't limit your freedom.

If he does have feelings then he is unable or unwilling to express them. He repeats the refrain 'What you see is what there is' and takes enormous delight in batting back the speculations and interpretations of those who attempt to find out what hides behind the deliberately wacky, nomadic, wise-cracking, non-stop chatting image.

Faced with what appears to be a non-existent love life, some interviewers have speculated darkly on skeletons in the closet. Lynn Barber, in a newspaper interview published just before mine, went so far as to confront him with the rumour that he likes little girls. He rubbished that with his characteristic patter. With me, he declares quite coldly that he actually doesn't like children very much at all. I was inclined to believe him and to believe too that he doesn't much care for the patients at Broadmoor, the sick at St James's, the physically disabled at Stoke Mandeville or the hundreds and thousands of other people and causes he helps by virtue of his publicity, his marathon running, his Jim'll fix it approach. This is no Mother Teresa spirtually ministering to people's emotional and material needs. Jimmy Savile says he is what you see. If he is to be believed then he is a calculating materialist who does what he does because that is what gives him the greatest sense of control, freedom, independence. He does not need people. But he can cope with people who need him as long as they are satisfied with the things he is prepared and able to give them – in most instances material things, in no instance himself.

He is indeed a man with a knack for making money and it is a knack that has served many a cause well. I doubt that any of them will worry too much that the precise cause matters little to Jimmy Savile 'whether it's a fish and chip shop or a church'. Why should it? He undertakes to raise the funds required and he is more often than not as good as his word. His achievements are astonishing, the very stuff of legend. In over twenty years of campaigning, this man has raised over £30 million. But he is certainly interesting and, in my experience, different in this one regard. It is of course true that many people who are active in what might be called charitable works are there by accident rather than design. For every campaigner for a cause who is personally affected or knows a relative or friend who is affected, there are many more who are active in this or that particular cause merely because they were asked. But it is uncommon in my experience for activists however recruited to maintain quite the same degree of disinterest as is manifested by Savile in his discussion of Stoke Mandeville or Broadmoor Hospital.

After the interview I recall asking him about his brothers and sisters all of who have married and have forty-eight children between them. Once again, his comments somehow came around to money. Feelings do indeed seem to baffle him. There is an exchange in the interview between us over the issue of marriage. Stung by my asking him why he remains unmarried, he challenges me to give him a reason why he should be? I suggest the desire to share, love and the wish to have the loved one with you. He bluntly replies that he does not know what love is and then embarks on a seemingly obfuscating passage on the various definitions of love available. But I don't believe it is obfuscating. In fact it is quite revealing. Perhaps he hasn't encountered love, he suggests, because he was 'too business-like' – and once again there is the emphasis on material things, possessions, achievements, security. Perhaps too calculating – the implication here is the emotions lead you astray, are dangerous, cause trouble. Perhaps it is that he has always felt that the grass over the hill is greener – his reluctance to plant emotional roots is mirrored in his refusal to identify any one physical location as home. His choice of the term 'pirate' to describe himself seems exceedingly apt.

When the recording of the interview with Sir James Savile OBE ended it was late in the evening. I remember that I had to return to my own family and was anxious to do so but he appeared in no hurry to go. He relaxed a little and chafed me as to what I had got out of it. I parried by observing that if what he chooses to reveal is what there is and all that there is then the listeners would be in a rare position to answer the question that people so often ask, namely what is Jimmy Savile really like? He is certainly a very bright man, nobody's fool, quick, sharp, witty and in control. He has that common and contrary mixture of respect and contempt for those who have had higher education of a formal kind and he sets in the balance their cleverness and his common sense. His common sense wins out not least because it causes less problems.

To date he appears a reasonably contented man but how can one tell? Maybe it is my doubts that I could or would be able to live his pirate life that push me to project into him a foreboding that his solitary, shifting life is but a manifestation of a profound psychological malaise with its roots in that materially deprived, emotionally somewhat indifferent childhood which he so flatly describes. There is something chilling about this twentieth-century 'saint' which still intrigues me to this day. No, not an easy interview but, for me at any rate, not a forgettable one either.

CLARE: Sir James Wilson Savile OBE was born on October 31st 1926, the youngest of seven children. His father was a bookmaker's clerk, his mother in her teenage a teacher. A Roman Catholic, James left school at fourteen to work in an office, later in the South Yorkshire coalfield, but an injury finished a budding career as a coal-miner. In the early 1950s he commenced his career as the country's first disc jockey, in Leeds and then with the Mecca organisation in London. In 1957 he joined Radio Luxemburg and while there took up wrestling and fought over a hundred fights. He compered the first performance of *Top of the Pops* at six o'clock on Wednesday, January 1st 1964. His radio and TV achievements, together with his remarkable and highly successful work for charity were marked by an award of an OBE in 1970. In 1975 *Jim'll Fix It* began on BBC 1 and sixteen years later is running still. In 1980 he was made a Knight of St Gregory by the Pope and in 1990 he was knighted by the Queen.

Now Jimmy Savile, I saw you quoted, perhaps inaccurately that psychiatrists should be burned. Why did you agree to this interview?

SAVILE: Because I agree to everything. I might have done a lot and I might have learned a lot but I still haven't learnt to say no, yet.

CLARE: You find that very difficult.

SAVILE: Yes, very difficult, yes, yes, I actually get enthusiastic over things because if somebody comes to me with a problem I finish up getting far more enthusiastic over their problems than they do and it's a terrible habit, it's terrible and it involves you in monumental problems yourself. The only problems I ever get personally are other people's, I don't have any of my own.

CLARE: Is it related to a fear of hurting other people? That by saying no . . .

SAVILE: I've tried to analyse it and it could be for instance that maybe I'm not clever enough to have problems, I don't, my mind doesn't allow problems to lurk in my head, so if somebody else comes to me with one it could be the fact that it might be intriguing.

CLARE: Does the fact that you feel you have no problems mean that you're a happy man?

SAVILE: Oh, totally, yes, yes totally.

CLARE: Do you ever get depressed?

SAVILE: Not really, no, no, not really.

CLARE: You've seen people get depressed?

SAVILE: I've seen people take their lives with depression. I've helped people with depression for many many years, not because I want to, it's just because if you come up against somebody that has a problem, we'll say depression, then you will talk to them because in this world there are not all that many people who have the inclination or the time to actually listen to somebody else's problem. In my general hospitals where I was a voluntary helper, like Leeds Infirmary or Stoke Mandeville, patients are constantly surprised that I might actually finish up pulling up a chair and sitting down by the bed and say 'Well what did you think about before you went down to the operation and you said you were worried about . . .?' Nobody ever talks to them like that and of course they feel terrific then. Now I don't do it to make them feel terrific.

I do it because I get quite interested in the way that their head's working.

CLARE: Because you apparently never get depressed, does it intrigue you that other people get depressed? Is it understandable to you? Do you understand why others would get low?

SAVILE: It intrigues me, but not to the point where I want to know why they get depressed. It will make me sad for them that they get depressed and I know that one thing you don't say to depressed people is pull yourself together. But there are times when you have to say pull yourself together but you have to know when to say it, you see. It's very intriguing. Whereas some people are interested in Georgian silver and some people are interested in butterflies, I was always interested in people, 'cos when I was very very young, being the youngest of seven, I had big ears and no mouth because nobody listens to you when you're the youngest of a family anyway so you finish up listening a lot. I used to think how strange this person was from that person and then I'd listen to the folks or brothers and sisters talking about them afterwards and it all went into a big jumble of a computer. We didn't have any money for hobbies of any sort so it would appear, I don't know, but it would appear that people finished up almost as a hobby.

CLARE: For you?

SAVILE: Yes.

CLARE: It sounds as if you were a happy child?

SAVILE: Well I wasn't unhappy because we didn't have anything and if you didn't have anything and you weren't expecting anything, and I've tried to analyse my childhood and wonder why when one had nothing and one expected nothing did that mean that one was happier? I think it's for somebody else but let me try this on you, seeing as I'm working for you for nothing you can work for me for nothing. Now in my early youth which was, we'll say I would be anything from seven, eight, ten years of age – which is an impressionable age and you see more than you let on and that you realise that you see – at Christmas time the big deal in our house – I keep harping on about no money but if there's no money there's no money you understand, so there's no big presents or anything like that – the big thrill was to go down to a department store in Leeds which had just opened in those days and look around that which we'd never seen before, which was the toy fair or the toy floor. And there was this vast area, this enormous area with toys, all flashed up and things like that and it was like an Aladdin's cave. Now analysing it I never went in expecting one of them. It never occurred to me that we could actually come out with one. In actual fact, on reflection, it could have been that had I brought one out, it would have lost its glamour and glitter. In its setting it was terrific. It was marvellous to go down there, to walk around and see all these amazing things. And then the big deal came because they used to have large paper cups of orangeade for three old pence, it's like half a pence now or whatever it is, and we'd finish up, the Duchess would buy me one of those – I call my mother the Duchess 'cos she costs me as much as one – but that was phenomenal. Now today I understand, I'm not quite sure, but I understand that if a kid looks at the TV and he sees a new toy on TV the kid will automatically wonder how he will or she will actually acquire one. It never occurred to me to acquire anything.

CLARE: Would that have been true for the other six in your family?

SAVILE: Not necessarily because you see with me I think the folks ran out of steam. I was what I've come to call a 'not-again child.' Now a 'not-again child' is when the Duchess told all her chinas that she was up the tub, they'd say 'Not again!' you see. So I finished up as a not-again child, so I wasn't really budgeted for.

CLARE: Did you ever sense as a child that your parents had mixed feelings about your arrival?

SAVILE: No, no, no, no they didn't have any feelings. It was complete equanimity insofar as I was there and that's all there was to it. And there was another mouth, there was six mouths to feed so the difference between six and seven wasn't even one.

CLARE: What was the difference in age between the eldest and you?

SAVILE: I don't know. We're all still alive, thank God, and we all love each other and all have great fun with each other. I don't know. My eldest brother and sister they're about a hundred I think, I'm not sure, but I mean they were vastly older than me, they still are vastly older than me!

CLARE: All in Britain?

SAVILE: One's in Australia, we sold one but yes, they're all around, all carrying on.

CLARE: And you all had good relationships with each other?

SAVILE: Sure, it was a big family, big love-ins, big fall-outs like any other big robust family.

CLARE: What was your father like?

SAVILE: The old man, he was marvellous, he was marvellous. My only regret, one of my few regrets, is that he never lived long enough to see a few of my quid. The Duchess had sixteen years of plenty of money.

CLARE: What age were you when he died?

SAVILE: Oh, I don't know, I should think in my twenties maybe. You see I was still down the pit and still damaged when he was about. I would dearly love, have loved to have had him around because you know you have your folks and they like what you've done etc. etc. But I missed all that with him but I got plenty of it with the Duchess.

CLARE: How close were you to him?

SAVILE: As close as you could be. At that age you don't understand closeness, you don't understand closeness. You only understand closeness when you haven't got it. We had, looking back, a terrific relationship. He demanded nothing from me. I demanded nothing at all from him. We had this great communion and union as it were. We didn't have any particular hobbies as such, you know, we didn't go fishing or didn't have anything that cost anything.

CLARE: Did you know much about what he did?

SAVILE: No. The only thing I know was he never ever got up

before eleven o'clock in the morning 'cos the horse-racing didn't start till twelve. So we would be up and school and we had to sort of tippitoe about because him getting up was quite symbolic insofar as he'd get up at eleven o'clock. He'd spend about four hours in the bathroom and he would come downstairs and he would have tea with no milk and he would have a slice of bread and dripping and then he would walk off somewhere and I understood that it was something to do with horses. But of course it never occurred to me why people should put money on a horse or anything like that. He had not a bad life, getting up at eleven o'clock in the morning.

CLARE: Were there things about him that remind you now of yourself?

SAVILE: Not really, except he was a fella, I'm a fella. But I'm a pirate, he was never a pirate, he was too honest.

CLARE: What do you mean, a pirate?

SAVILE: Well I'm a pirate, I mean he was honest, he was lovely. He had a job. He went and stuck to it.

CLARE: Aren't you honest?

SAVILE: I'm 'dishonest' in inverted commas insofar as I'm a ducker and diver and if I see an opportunity of getting something by only going halfway round the course I'll do it unfortunately! When you're well known like me you never get round to being like that because there's too many people watching you! In other words if I've got to run twenty-six-point-two miles I've got to run twenty-six-point-two miles. I can't get in a taxi 'cos they'll say 'Where were you halfway round, you were missed?'

CLARE: But if you could you would? Are you a gambler?

SAVILE: No, no, no, no, no, no. You know when people swim they swim with their arms going outward? I can't swim but if I was to swim I would swim with my arms coming in 'cos I'd even gather the water in! I'm no gambler. I've no stocks, no shares, no nothing. What I've got nobody else ever sees. It never sees the light of day. If I pulled a ten pound note out now the Queen's eyes would blink against the light, because nobody ever sees what I've got. It's gone for all time!

CLARE: That isn't to suggest for a minute that you don't like it. You quite like, I take it, the trappings that go with fame – the money, the Rolls Royces, etc.?

SAVILE: Oh, I love it, love it. If I say they don't bother me they actually don't bother me. I got a Rolls Royce initially because I realised that in my line of business that I'd chosen which was a flash game, a posing game, a candy-floss game, a phenomenon . . .

CLARE: The disc jockey game?

SAVILE: Well the pop business . . . yes that was total phenomenon, total candy-floss, and I realised that if I had a Rolls Royce that it would make a difference. and it did. Because I lived in Yorkshire, I lived in Leeds and when I came to London for the Radio Luxemburg thing I was introduced as 'This is Jimmy Savile from Leeds. He has a Rolls.' And that made all the difference in the world you see. On the occasion I used to drive down in it it made a tremendous difference so I saw that as a tool of the trade, purely and simply.

CLARE: How early do you remember doing that, using things to make that kind of impact? You've done that over the years – the way you've dressed, your hairstyle, the language that you used in those early disc-jockey days. But how far back does one have to go to find you doing that? When did you find that if you adopted some oddity then people noticed you?

SAVILE: If you take the Rolls Royce, then when I was down the pit, I was in my teens then and I came across a picture of a Rolls Royce in a book, it was a black and white picture like a line drawing almost, but because it was the best of the best – even then I knew that something like a Rolls Royce was the best of the best – I actually cut the picture out and pinned it up inside my wardrobe. There was absolutely no chance me even seeing one, let alone owning one, so it could be – are you a psychologist or a psychiatrist?

CLARE: A psychiatrist.

SAVILE: A psychiatrist. Oh you've got chances. You do things with pills whereas psychologists do things with words.

CLARE: I do both really, yes.

SAVILE: So therefore you can tell me why it was I, at that age, pulled out that picture because you could then define possibly that there might have been something lurking that even I didn't know about. But a Rolls Royce, it was part ... I never got hooked on what I'd got, I never wanted to keep up with the Joneses, everything was a means to an end.

CLARE: Did you enjoy the Rolls Royce?

SAVILE: Loved it.

CLARE: You enjoyed sitting in it and driving it?

SAVILE: Oh yes, big posing job.

CLARE: You have a Rolls Royce now?

SAVILE: I've had seventeen new ones.

CLARE: What's so important about a new one?

SAVILE: Well, because my theory is this. Your qualifications will last you till your last breath, whereas I'm still in the phenomenon business. I can go skint in a day. I can be finished like that. If a scandal comes up or something like that or the people go off you, you're finished. I'd much rather go skint with a brand new Rolls Royce in the garage than one that's eight years old that I love, because I'll get more for it. So the day that I get finished by some whatever, then the bits and pieces that I've got I'll make sure that they're all paid up and they're all brand new because I could then go and be very unhappy in the South of France, covered in shame and sunshine and mad birds with bikinis on for a long time because there was a new Rolls Royce there and a new this and a new that. So I am all terribly logical which is actually bad news for you guys, because common sense and logic don't leave you with a lot to find out.

CLARE: No, we're much more interested in feelings, emotions ...

SAVILE: Yes, right, emotions, I haven't got any.

CLARE: Do you worry? Do you plan ahead?

SAVILE: Oh, aye.

CLARE: You said to me 'If there were a scandal.' You mean if somebody wrote something? What could they write disreputably about Jimmy Savile?

SAVILE: Oh, yes well they don't have to have a reason for

writing. I mean they can write for no reason. In actual fact today the concern has been taken away, not worry, the concern. I must explain to the listeners I'm talking funny now 'cos I've got a cigar in my face. I'll take it out and talk properly again. In the old days, we'll say ten years ago, many people were ruined in my game by scandals that never existed. It was just at the behest of somebody who wrote about them. Today it's not like that at all, because today we can actually sue people who tell lies. Ten years ago you couldn't do that, believe me and today it's OK because if anybody tells lies about us today that means we finish up with even more money and that'll do for me, so we've got even less to worry about.

CLARE: Have you ever had to sue?

SAVILE: Oh, aye, yes, yes I sued a couple of papers and they give me about thirty grand . . .

CLARE: Really, they libelled you?

SAVILE: Yes, marvellous.

CLARE: What did they say?

SAVILE: I don't know what they said. They said I'd said something which I hadn't and I'd ring up a brief and he says 'Leave it to me' and then he rings me back and he says 'They want to give you thirty grand' and I said 'The best of Irishman's luck to 'em, we'll have it,' and he said 'Terrific,' so suddenly I got thirty grand and thought this is a marvellous game is this. Ten years ago that could never have happened, because they could have said what they wanted and it would have been very very difficult to sue them. But along came somebody like Jeffrey Archer who got half a million pounds and Koo Stark who got a fortune of money, so all of a sudden unscruptulous newspaper people, they're not the norm, thank God, but there were plenty of them around in those days, they realised first of all it's now going to cost them a fortune, today it costs them their job as well.

CLARE: You mentioned logic in relation to your psychology and you say that's bad news for people like me because we're interested in irrationality, if you like, and oddity and emotional disturbance and stress.

SAVILE: Yes, I say that 'cos you people deal with patients you see. I'm an oddity because I'm not here for treatment. I have got awesome common sense and my common sense obviously works 'cos it's worked for me, that would make me bad news for a psychiatrist or a psychologist because there's nothing to find. What you see is what there is, so that's why I say I'm bad news for somebody like you. God forbid I should have a problem and I have to come and see you with a problem, then I'll be the same as everybody else.

CLARE: But the thing that tends to get us into difficulties are our feelings. They cannot be predicted or controlled.

SAVILE: No because you see feelings are not logic as such and feelings can come out of a box inside you anywhere. I mean they can suddenly pop out. I mean if you have a tendency to violence for instance.

CLARE: Now what about your feelings?

SAVILE: I haven't found them yet.

CLARE: Seriously.

SAVILE: No, I haven't found them yet. The only feelings I get is exhaustion when I've done about nineteen miles in a marathon or when I'm fed up if I'm on a train and I'm lumbered on a train and somebody that's got drunk at the bar recognises me . . . I mean they're all my best pals you understand.

CLARE: What about the feelings you had for your mother, the Duchess?

SAVILE: The Duchess. Yes well that was, yes that was something because I actually enjoyed the Duchess. I didn't enjoy it in the early days because you have to learn to enjoy your parents you see.

CLARE: Why? What was she like in the early days?

SAVILE: She was all right but obviously she would tell you to do things and you didn't particularly want to do them. She'd say I'm putting your board up next week, and I'd think that was terribly unfair, and all those usual sort of little things. But eventually when I came into a few quid and I suddenly realised that I could actually have a better time teaming her about with me than I could teaming a girl about with me, 'cos a girl would give me brain damage but the Duchess, we could have a meal, we could go somewhere. Very often I'd ring her up and say 'What are you doing?' and she'd say 'Nothing,' because the Duchess has this marvellous theory. She used to say to all my sisters 'Always be prepared to take your pinafore off and go out with your husband, because if you don't he'll soon find somebody who will.' So of course she practised what she preached. So if I rang up and said 'What are you doing? – nothing, right I'll be up in a minute.' I once took her to see the Pope and she was convinced that she was going to Jersey. And she said 'You don't want to say things like that,' she said, 'you'll get into trouble,' and we arrived in Rome and it was all quite amazing you see and we finished up at the wrong end of St Peter's Square. And she suddenly took over and came in front of me and barged through about half a million people and threatened a nine foot tall papal guard if he didn't let her in, 'cos she had a ticket to see the Pope, if he didn't let her in she would kill him you see! Of course when the Pope comes past in the chair and the Duchess was there doing the swooning job, all dressed in black with the lace and I'd never seen her look like that before, and she was going to be mortally disappointed if he didn't give her the ace, king, queen, jack and he looked down and I pointed to the Duchess – he gives her a smile and nodded head, oh a big swooning job! So I mean we had a great time, you couldn't have that time with a girl you see.

CLARE: Why?

SAVILE: Well because, because a girl would be a different kettle of fish, because a girl is much more of a partnership. As against the Duchess – she brought me up for the first part of my life and I brought her up for the second part of her life.

CLARE: A girl too would have expectations of you?

SAVILE: I haven't the faintest idea.

CLARE: A girl would make demands.

SAVILE: Oh, I don't know, I don't mind them making demands on me. Oh yes, ladies can demand me any time.

CLARE: But one of the demands they might make is that your life would be changed, that you couldn't be a pirate.

SAVILE: Really?

CLARE: I'm asking you.

SAVILE: I don't know. I'm not a girl. I can't tell you. You'll have to ask a girl about what she wants.

CLARE: Nonetheless you've never had one for any length of time.

SAVILE: Oh, yes, yes, some of the girls I know now I've known thirty, forty years, and some I've known thirty, forty minutes.

CLARE: But you've never married.

SAVILE: Oh, no, good heavens, no couldn't do that.

CLARE: Why not?

SAVILE: Why not? All right, I'll reverse it. You give me a good reason for getting married.

CLARE: Well often a reason would be to share one's life.

SAVILE: Now you're not all that confident now are you?

CLARE: No, because there are many reasons for getting married, as you know.

SAVILE: But I've never found a good one. Sure there's many reasons for getting married. Somebody puts a gun to your head.

CLARE: Well people get married because they're in love.

SAVILE: Really?

CLARE: Well, have you been?

SAVILE: Never.

CLARE: Never in love?

SAVILE: I don't know what it is.

CLARE: I suppose the best definition is that the person you're in love with, if she goes away you miss her and want her back.

SAVILE: Not if you're a pirate 'cos there's plenty where you're going.

CLARE: That's why I'm asking, has that ever happened to you?

SAVILE: No, not yet, no.

CLARE: Have many of your brothers and sisters married?

SAVILE: Oh yes they're all married, they're all nice and normal and skint.

CLARE: Why were you different?

SAVILE: I haven't the faintest idea, maybe it was the 'not-again' one.

CLARE: Did any of them have a large family?

SAVILE: Oh, aye, one of my sisters has got fourteen children.

CLARE: What does she make of you?

SAVILE: She's got enough for fourteen, she doesn't bother with me. She loves me 'cos we get on dead well together.

CLARE: What do you think you had for your mother, was that love?

SAVILE: No. You see the word 'love' is only one word in the English language, 'love.' In the Greek there are about fifty-seven words meaning love. In Greek there's the love of a tree, there's the love of a lake, love of a drink, love of food. It's a different word, and that's why they always say 'The Greeks have a word for it.' Now the word that leaves your mouth which is love in the meaning in your brain is not necessarily the meaning in my brain when I catch the ball that you've just thrown to me you see, 'cos we have only one word. I will try to help and I will say I know what you're saying in relation to love and marriage but I'm saying that that particular route wasn't one that attracted me, not that I'm funny or weird or anything like that. Maybe if I try to analyse why I didn't, maybe I was too business-like, maybe I was too calculating, maybe I was too much of a pirate, maybe the view over the hill might have been better than the view I'd got. I don't know, you would have to tell me. All I know is that today might be whatever it is, Monday, Tuesday, Wednesday, Thursday, I don't even know what day it is, and that's all I'm positive of. I'm not positive of tomorrow, I don't know what tomorrow's going to bring and I'm quite happy that up to press everything's OK. And I don't see it no big deal that I didn't ever get wed.

CLARE: What about being lonely?

SAVILE: No. Being alone and lonely are two different things. I'm often alone because I purposely will go training over the moors in Yorkshire, or in Scotland or wherever because to be under God's sky with a reasonable temperature or even an unreasonable temperature you have been blessed to such an extent because you're body's working like an oiled thing and you're saying to it run up this hill at the same speed as you ran down the other side and things like that. Now there's a certain animalistic pleasure in that, so I quite love being alone. By the same rule if somebody suddenly appears out of a hole in the ground and says 'I'll run with you,' I'll say 'Terrific,' so it doesn't matter to me if I've got people or I haven't got people.

CLARE: No, so you certainly like being alone or with people. You don't feel lonely or feel the need for someone to confide in particularly.

SAVILE: No, you see let me try something else on you. I have friends who, who are married, right. They got married nice and young we'll say, they're married. Now then they finish up saying to themselves that the punter they've got is not the right punter, right. So they want to leave the punter. They apparently can't wait and they can't leave. And this applies to men as well as women. They can't leave that one till they've organised the next one you see and there's no gap in between one and the other. Now personally I do find that a bit strange as it happens, I mean out of the frying pan into the frying pan. You know it's a bit strange, but if that's the way they want it that's them not me. So that I should act like that would be totally foreign to me and I reserve the right to think that it's amazing that they must have another one lined up before they leave the first one, as though they're panic-stricken or something to be on their own. Me, to be on my own I'd give a few quid to be on my own sometimes. I once walked from John O'Groats to Lands End to be on my own and I was never on my own any one of the thirty-one days, the punters all came out and walked with me.

CLARE: What about children?

SAVILE: Yes, I couldn't eat a whole one.

CLARE: Do you like children?

SAVILE: Hate them.

CLARE: Really, seriously?

SAVILE: That's why I get on well with them, 'cos I don't like them all that much. A kid with me is on trial, like I'm on trial with the kid, you know what I mean? If you come to a kid and you want to impress the kid you've got a tough job on. So the kid's on trial with me, so it's like a stand off. Now instinctively the kid knows that I ain't like some yukky adult that says 'My don't you look smart today?' or any crap like that, you know what I mean? I'll say 'Hello. Here I am, with this TV show called *Jim'll Fix It* and you're on it so therefore you have to earn the right to be on it. Answer me question' and the kid will answer me question and we got on like a house on fire but there's no yukky nonsense about it and I've got no paternal feelings. So if you said to me 'What about kids?' I say basically I don't think I like them particularly, but I get on well with them. Nothing wrong with that is there?

CLARE: Not a thing, no.

SAVILE: Here, halfway, I mean to say from what you were talking am I weird or am I ordinary or what?

CLARE: I'll tell you at the end.

SAVILE: Oh, all right then.

CLARE: Do you think people think you are weird?

SAVILE: Well, I suppose it's rather like if you got five people on a panel to judge the Miss World Competition, the five judges will give you a one, two, three. If you got five other people, totally different people, they'd give you a different one, two, three. It's in the eyes of the beholder. It bothers me to an extent but not particularly 'cos I do my thing. All I check with myself is 'Am I offending anybody? Am I upsetting anybody? Am I being unreasonable?' or whatever and if the answer to those are all good answers then I do my thing. Now if anybody gets the wrong end of the stick, well that's hard luck. And because there's six thousand million people on this earth you're bound to get somebody who'll get the wrong end of the stick, so it ain't no big deal.

CLARE: When you say it bothers you to some extent . . .

SAVILE: Well, yes because we wouldn't get washed in a morning if we weren't bothered about what people thought of us. You know, we wouldn't put our clothes in the washing

machine, we'd stink and we'd go round like the Neanderthal
people did but we don't do that 'cos we're developed to a
degree, so therefore we obviously must regard what people
think of us otherwise we wouldn't put colourful clothes on
or whatever.

CLARE: Do you ever think you are odd or unusual?

SAVILE: Oh yes unusual, yes because I'm not like, right, fifty-
five million people in this country, I'm not like a lot of them.
Therefore I must be an odd person out, but odd in that sense
is only a numerical odd, it is not necessarily an odd odd . . .

CLARE: When you started out, it sounds as if very cold-
bloodedly, logically, you made yourself outrageous. In a
cutting I saw that you changed the colour of your hair I
think from show to show on *Top of the Pops*. You knew it
would make a point.

SAVILE: No. It was all a laugh, and it all started for a laugh
insofar as I'm in my dancehall minding my own business,
playing the records, a lad comes up to me, he said 'Here why
don't you come to our hairdressing salon?' And I said 'What
on earth do I want to come to a hairdressing salon for?' And
he said 'There's five floors and it's full of girls' and I said 'I'll
be there tonight.' And I walked in because they were having
a students night, you see and they said 'So what do we do?'
and I said 'I don't know.' And I looked around, I'd never
been in a ladies hairdressing salon before and I said 'Make
me blonde.' So they said 'Yes, all right.' So they slapped
some stuff on my head that took the top of my head off, and
I finished up a raving blonde, went back to the dancehall
and it brought the place to a grinding halt. I mean people
screamed and carried on and rushed up to the front of the
stage, and there was nobody more amazed than me. Why
would they want to perform like that just 'cos one minute
my hair was dark, the next minute it's light? Then here
comes the business take-over. I thought 'Crikey, if we get
that sort of reaction, wow, hey we're in business here. We've
discovered a gimmick,' 'cos in those days, in the sixties,
gimmicks were the thing, and gimmicks make the difference
between getting a Rolls Royce and not getting a Rolls Royce.

Or getting some money and feeling comfortable or going back to being skint like I was. And in those days I didn't want to be skint, 'cos I didn't want the Duchess should go back with me into the lifestyle that we'd left. So I was concerned about keeping up the level of income because she was my only outgoing as it were and I took unto myself the fact that I quite enjoyed looking after her for the second half of her life. So when I found a gimmick like that then I milked it for all it was worth and it paid. It was like putting money in a jackpot machine and you get a jackpot every time you pull the handle. Nothing wrong with that, business is business.

CLARE: This interest you have, this enormous interest you have in charity, the amounts of money you've raised for charity . . .

SAVILE: May I correct you? I haven't really got an interest in charity, not really.

CLARE: Raising money, I should say, for all sorts of causes . . .

SAVILE: Not really, no it's just that I've got a knack, I think you're putting the cart before the horse there. Because I've got a knack for raising money or making money now, I don't really care whether I make it . . .

CLARE: Yes, but you don't just make it for yourself.

SAVILE: No, I don't care whether I make it for me or somebody else, it's academic to me, as long as I'm having a go at making it.

CLARE: But you make it for Stoke Mandeville and not as far as I know for the British Aircraft Corporation.

SAVILE: Ah, because I went to Stoke Mandeville twenty-four years ago to give some prizes away. I got caught up with the job that they're doing and I've been there ever since. I went to Broadmoor twenty-four years ago again to give some prizes away, got caught up with the enormous task that the staff have to do there, almost impossible tasks and I've stayed there ever since. Now I had no axe to grind. I get many people, you know, come to me and they say 'I want to tell you about . . .' and they'll mention an illness. The fact that I could lecture on the illness, they don't even check on that, and I'll listen to them, then I'll say 'Which one of your family has got it?' 'Well it's my brother, sister, auntie, uncle . . .' and I say 'Would you be as interested in it if your brother, sister, auntie, uncle didn't have it?' Now that is almost an unkind thing to say and I don't usually say that, but in my mind I say that, because they have a vested interest. I haven't got a vested interest in any one of the, as it were, charities that I look after, none whatsoever.

CLARE: So how do you decide?

SAVILE: First come, first served.

CLARE: First come, first served?

SAVILE: First come, first served.

CLARE: Whoever gets your ears?

SAVILE: It matters little to me whether it's a fish and chip shop or a church.

CLARE: So the way you describe yourself, an awful lot of your life is as a result of things happening to you. You don't necessarily initiate these things.

SAVILE: I've never initiated anything, to my knowledge I've never ever initiated anything at all. Do you know, I've never asked for a job in my life, ever. Never, I mind my own business, the phone goes, or I get a letter, bingo I'm off again.

CLARE: The world's first disc jockey — how did that come about? Was that in any sense initiated by you?

SAVILE: It was about nineteen forty-four and I'd been injured in a mine explosion — I was working as a miner — and I couldn't do anything and I couldn't earn a living and I'd heard of one of my pals who'd contrived to fasten the inside of a valve radio to the pick-up arm of a wind-up gramophone, and the noise came out of the radio instead of coming out of the gramophone, which was unreal, I mean ooee! I shuffled round with my two sticks, have a listen to this, and borrowed it off him, wrote out some tickets, 'cos I suddenly had this great flash and I thought 'This is it, it's a band' but like you know, the best band from America and I wrote these tickets out, 'Grand Record Dance — One Shilling' and I sold eleven tickets you see and they all turned up and we put this equipment on top of a grand piano and it lasted forty minutes because the wires, the bare wires inbetween glowed red hot and charred the top of the piano and they melted at the soldered joints. Nobody asked for their money back because it was a brave attempt you see and people said 'What a pity.' Now they saw it as a disaster. I saw it differently. At the time I was getting seventy-five pence a week sick money and I'd suddenly got eleven bob. The room was ten shillings fifty pence but the man says 'It's all right, it's all right, it wasn't your fault' so nobody wanted any money off me. And I got eleven bob, in forty minutes! Do me a favour, had to work seven days for seventy-five pence! And at that point a girl comes up and she said 'Will it ever work, this stuff?' and I said 'Oh, yes, it'll work next time.' She said 'Good it's my twenty-first. I can't afford a band. How much do you charge?' And I said 'Two pound ten' and she gave me an address and she said 'Will you bring it up?' and so I got my pal to make up a more robust one and the world's first live disc jockey was held in a room in Ottley in Yorkshire and the audience was from two to eighty-two and I plugged the thing into the wall and it worked all night with about nine records and I played both sides of them over and over again. I got something to eat. I got a girl to walk home, chatted up a girl to walk home, and it was such a marvellous night I forgot to get paid and the girl whose birthday it was came rushing back in. She said 'Here, I forgot to pay you.' I went 'Oh, yes.' And she put two pound notes and a ten bob note in my hand and I looked at it and I thought 'I'm a millionaire!' I'm nine point nine hundred thousand and odd short at that precise moment, but I knew I was a millionaire, like with a million pounds because I had to be a millionaire because it was that easy and that was it. There wasn't one before that pal, there just wasn't.

CLARE: But that you did initiate. You saw the possibilities.

SAVILE: No, it was my pal that invented it. All I did was see the possibility of a machine. So I only came in halfway along really.

CLARE: You're a man who finds it difficult to say no.

SAVILE: Unfortunately, yes.

CLARE: What if a woman asked you to marry her?

SAVILE: I will find it very easy to say no!

CLARE: You once described yourself as an archetypal single man.

SAVILE: Yes. I'm not quite sure what archetypal means but it sounded OK.

CLARE: What would you say are the features that make you ideal as a single man?

SAVILE: I like being on my own. I like climbing into bed on my own, and I like being able to do exactly what I want to do, when I want to do it. And now of course the ultimate luxury is that I've got all the money that was ever printed. I think I've got nearly a full set of white fivers, as it happens. You can do what you want when you want, and it is all too much. And so all the concerns that I had, like when the Duchess was alive, going skint, things like that, I haven't got any of those concerns now. So I just breeze along and all I have to make sure is that I'm not turning into a pain in the arse or smug to people or anything like that.

CLARE: Are you ever distressed?

SAVILE: Only when I see how unfortunate life can be for some other poor sod who doesn't deserve what life deals out to him, but hang on, I don't know that tomorrow isn't my turn. It hasn't been my turn up to press. One of my patients at Stoke Mandeville, bless her, is over eighty. Now at eighty there's this nice lady who thought 'Am I alive?' when she wakes up in the morning 'cos when you're eighty you start to think like that, right? And she tripped over the chord of her Hoover and she broke her neck and she has to learn all over again, living you see. Now I'm not eighty yet, you're not eighty yet, a lot of the listeners aren't eighty yet – don't get too clever folks, 'cos you don't know what's round the corner. So you make sure today you've got plenty of compassion, you've got plenty of time for compassion for people, 'cos you don't know if your turn comes tomorrow, I don't know if my turn comes tomorrow but up to press I've had a marvellous time.

CLARE: When you mother's turn came, was that expected or unexpected?

SAVILE: What, when she died? Oh, totally unexpected. She taught me a great lesson in dying. She was very concerned that she was going to be a burden to people, you know old people of the old school are like that, 'cos in the old days you could be a real burden to people. And she worried about it you see and I couldn't worry about it, because she wasn't a burden so therefore I didn't know what she was worrying about. When she decided to die she did it all in twenty minutes and in twenty minutes she gave the great honour of dying to one of my sisters (she happened to be in one of my sisters' house for the weekend) and she said 'Get a priest and a doctor.' They were just going to bed you see and my sister says 'What?' She said 'Get a priest and a doctor.' So what the Duchess said you did. So my sister got a priest and a doctor there and then. Within twenty minutes they were round, because my sister flapped a bit to think that maybe you know things weren't right. And the priest came round, the doctor came round. It was, it was almost scripted and she pegged it in twenty minutes and so for me, apart from it being a disaster, it was one of those inevitable disasters that had to come so I was half ready for it even though there were no signs of it.

CLARE: She hadn't been ill?

SAVILE: No, she hadn't been ill at all. What did occur to me was that she had wasted a lot of her time worrying for years over being a burden when she needn't have worried all that time. So I thought to myself I don't worry about what's going to happen to me, but like I said to the ladies and gentlemen listening earlier, don't get too clever because we don't know what tomorrow brings, so give plenty of time for compassion for other people.

CLARE: There was an interesting reference to you and the death of your mother I saw somewhere. You said the five days that you spent with her after she was dead were the happiest days of your life. That may have been a misquote, I don't know.

SAVILE: Well, yes, yes, words are clumsy things, as you well know. You're in the game where people give you words and you have to analyse not what they said but what they mean. So therefore in this particular case she was gone. I accepted she was gone. She was in heaven. That was marvellous. She had no worries now, tremendous. She wasn't a burden to anybody like she was worried about, everything's marvellous, OK. So if she was happy, I was happy. We hadn't put her away yet and there she was lying around so to me they were good times. They were not the best times. I'd much rather that she hadn't died, but it was inevitable, therefore it had to be. Once upon a time I had to share her with a lot of people. We had marvellous times. But when she was dead she was all mine, for me. So therefore it finished up right, you understand, and then we buried her and that was that. That's the end of that. And one day, according to one's faith, my faith, being a Catholic lad, there is apparently I'm told a strong chance that we'll all meet up again. Well that'll do for me. But I'll have to take a few quid with me because she was always boning me for a few quid 'cos she was a pirate as well. I turned her into a pirate. She invented ghost pay-rolling. Do you know what ghost pay-rolling is? Ghost pay-rolling is creating people that don't exist that she pays but they don't exist and I pay her. She didn't pay anybody. It's called ghost pay-rolling.

CLARE: She was like you was she?

SAVILE: No she wasn't to start with but I made her like me. Oh yes, I brought her up for the second half of her life and I turned her into a pirate.

CLARE: What was she like?

SAVILE: She was the country's only eighty-six-year-old female gangster.

CLARE: But as your mother, when you were growing up, what was she like?

SAVILE: Perfectly ordinary. She had no money. She had another six to go at and my dad.

CLARE: Was she a very practical, unromantic womamn?

SAVILE: No, no, she wasn't practical at all. I suppose in her heart of hearts, if I look back and analyse it, she was wondering how the hell she got into such a situation. And if she'd had her chance all over again one thing she wouldn't have had was seven kids.

CLARE: Was she physically very affectionate?

SAVILE: No, no. There was no tactile affection. If you were not well then there would be constant attention and things like that but we are not a tactile family. We don't rush and put our arms round each other and things like that. We just say 'Hello, how are you doing?' and it's just one of those natures that we are.

CLARE: Yes, and that's the way you all were with each other?

SAVILE: And still are, yes. If I suddenly leapt on and put my arms round a family member, they'd think I'm going round the bend, they'd probably give me a Beecham's powder!

CLARE: It sounds a reasonably tough survival – being the youngest of seven?

SAVILE: Not really, no when I come to look back. I didn't see anything about it that was tough at all. In comparison to somebody who had everything I suppose it could have been considered tough, but if you didn't have anything to start with you didn't realise it was tough.

CLARE: Was it a devout family? You say you were Roman Catholics.

SAVILE: Yes, not very devout at all. My dad never went to Mass. The Duchess did. My brothers and sisters did and they didn't. They did when they had to.

CLARE: Did you go to Catholic schools?

SAVILE: Yes we went to Catholic schools. But when I came to start working things out for myself I decided that I liked church like I like children! I can take it or leave it you understand. But I think it's not a bad thing. Kids aren't a bad thing really. Take them or leave them. Church is about the same. I go to Mass when I'm in London for instance. It's very handy because there's Mass at lunchtime or at six o'clock in the evening when I'm in London and so I can usually catch one or the other. And I actually like just going to Mass. I'm on me own at the back doing my own thing. I'm not quite sure why I'm there, but I know that it quite pleases me, so I do it.

CLARE: Is it something you think about much, your own death?

SAVILE: No I couldn't care less. When my time comes it comes.

CLARE: Or how you die?

SAVILE: Oh, yes, how you die is a bit important yes. I mean you don't want to be all messy and sticky and all carry on and hurtful. I'd much rather it come like that and that was it.

CLARE: Does it matter to you whether there's an afterlife?

SAVILE: I would hope that there would be, but if you were to say to me what is your definition of Christianity I would say that if you assured me that there was no afterlife, and that when you're dead that was that, then I would still do the things that I do for various charities and hospitals and things like that 'cos I don't do it particularly for reward. I once heard a monk on a radio programme and they said 'If it was proved there was no heaven would you stay in this monastery?' and he says 'Not two minutes.' I thought that was a bit odd because there's this marvellous fella, who obviously was living this life for some reward, and I thought that was a bit off personally.

CLARE: So you'd go on doing what you're doing. Would anything be affected by the revelation that there was nothing after death?

SAVILE: No, not in the slightest, not at all, wouldn't bother me.

CLARE: What does your faith give you?

SAVILE: Instinctively it gives me a nice feeling when I go to Mass. It's rather like that I've left the mad world outside and I've put a brake on all the things that don't matter like money and cars, and fame and stuff like that, and the things that do matter which is, am I heading in the right direction, am I doing the right thing for people and stuff like that. If I've been lucky am I really looking over my shoulder and giving somebody a pull up the path of life that's finding it a bit tougher than me? That to me is important, and when you get into church you can reflect on things like that that might be a bit difficult if you're sitting reflecting in a traffic jam on the M1 for instance.

CLARE: Would it be true to say that you have no close personal relationships with anyone, does anybody really know you very well?

SAVILE: You're in the business, you tell me.

CLARE: But in your judgement, do you think you have?

SAVILE: In my judgement?

CLARE: Is there somebody you'd say 'He or she knows me very well?'

SAVILE: I say 'What you see is what there is.' Now if what there is is acceptable so be it. If it's boring so be it, I can't help it, 'cos what there is is what there is. I'm sure that there are people who are close to me insofar as if I have helped somebody, we'll say for instance getting over a bad time or if I've helped somebody not die or whatever or whatever, they can become quite attached to you, now that's perfectly OK. I mean I've got patients who we've gone through some tough times together, and they're all right. Now I'm sure that maybe they might feel differently to me than I feel for them. I quite like them. My problem is I like everybody and it sounds a very yukky thing to say but unfortunately I'm stuck with it, I start off liking everybody, they've got to work a bit hard to make me not like them.

CLARE: So what I see is what you are and in that sense everybody who sees you knows you as much as they're ever likely to know you?

SAVILE: But they know me very well 'cos that's all there is to know. I mean I don't go away from here and indulge in some wild fetishes or wild weirdo things or anything like that. I mean, if you turned my stone over there ain't nothing underneath it. It's probably a boring stone for somebody like you who wants to find things out about people. What you're seeing is actually what there is, full stop.

CLARE: I would then hazard a guess that other people not knowing that what they see is what there is, will attempt to get to know you better. They'll be interested in what you think, what you feel.

SAVILE: That's all right by me. It's all right by them. Shall I tell you a quick story about this sort of thing, that happened about twenty years ago? A very famous professor of a very famous psychology department of a very famous university in this country got the same kick as you and he said 'I want to talk to that Savile,' he says ''cos he sounds a bit interesting,' not realising that what he saw was what there was. So Granada Television said 'Here, we could do a TV show. You go and analyse him and then you come on TV and tell us what makes him tick.' So the fellow said 'Terrific.' And he had three goes, three separate times. First of all in the studio, in a dressing room for about an hour and a half's tape and it ran out, and then he says 'No,' he says, 'I haven't got it,' he says. 'I want to go somewhere.' He'll come to a disco. And we went behind some doors so there wasn't too much noise and he thought it'd be different, and he had a go there. 'No, no, no,' he says, 'I want to go somewhere else.' All right, so three goes he had and by this time the TV producer was climbing up the wall you see and this man was a very famous professor. I can't tell you who he is 'cos he's still around. And the TV man says 'But you haven't got anything.' And he says 'No.' And then this professor leaned back and said 'I'd like my final year psychology students to have a go at this man.' So I said 'That's all right.' And the professor said 'Oh no it's not,' he says, 'because I want them to go out in the world thinking they stand a chance!'

CLARE: So, the moral of this story is that if we search for something inside you we will not find anything.

SAVILE: You've got to tell me, that's your game. I don't know. All I know is what I know. I mean you tell me. I mean I said to you 'Am I weird?' You got to tell me. I don't think I am, but I mean you're a specialist at your game and you could say 'You are the most weird person I've ever seen.' I say 'Terrific,' I'll get up and stick a cigar in my face, go out, jump in the Rolls Royce and bugger off.

CLARE: Well, I am intrigued, yes. Let me ask you and I'll tell you why I'm so interested in this area in a minute. It's not to do with sex so much as love. Has anybody fallen in love with you?

SAVILE: You better ask them.

CLARE: I've got to ask you.

SAVILE: All right. I don't know.

CLARE: Why do you say I better ask them? Somebody would have said it to you, would have said 'Jimmy, I love you.'

SAVILE: Oh, yes, a lot of people, a lot of ladies. Yes, nothing wrong with that. That's their problem, not mine.

CLARE: What is it that stops you there? That's where you do say no.

SAVILE: No 'cos that's not my game, that's not my lifestyle. The lifestyle that they want is just not my lifestyle.

CLARE: The key feature of your lifestyle is your control of it. You are master of your lifestyle. Nobody makes demands on your lifestyle. Such demands made are demands that you have in a sense accepted. You don't have any children. They make demands. You don't have a spouse that makes demands. You don't have close friends that make those kind of demands.

SAVILE: If anybody makes demands they don't make them twice pal because they get the sack after the first time.

CLARE: You do what you want to do.

SAVILE: Yes. I start off minding my own business. If anybody swims into my lifestyle and they want me to change they've had it, 'cos I won't, 'cos I can't. So they have to swim out again or stand back from me. What you see is what there is. One of the great problems of human relationships which you'll probably agree with me is that either one or other of the parties wants the other party to change, now I don't mean compromise, I don't mean all those things, I mean actually change and it doesn't work out.

CLARE: When you say what you see is what there is, you could say that in several ways. You could say, I mean a depressed person would say 'What you see is what there is and goddamn it, it doesn't amount to much!'

SAVILE: Ah, well, now then . . .

CLARE: And some rather grandiose person would say 'What you see is what there is and it's bloody good mate.'

SAVILE: Oh, no, I'd feel sorry for both of those people. Here is something that'll make the listeners easy to understand. I grew up in a phenomenal business, called the pop business, that was awash with booze and drugs. It never occurred to me to try either because I'm teetotal and I wouldn't even know what a drug looked like if I fell over it, right, because I was totally clear in my own mind that that wasn't my game. So 'cos it wasn't my game, I wasn't even tempted to have even a little dabble at it. As it happens I could see the terrible effects of what happened to people who did have a dabble at it, and I thought that was, from where I stood, quite stupid. But I didn't know what caused them to have a go at drugs or booze or whatever so let them get on with it, do you understand, it was nothing to do with me but I was right in the middle. I invented the disco game but it never occurred to me to go down the road of being stupid and foolish about it. Now if that's confidence from where you sit so be it, I call it common sense.

CLARE: Yes, OK. I would then guess, but you'll say well maybe maybe not, I don't know, I would guess at being the youngest of the seven in your case it gave you a certain space, a certain independence. There was a lot going on in your family but in a large family one of the advantages sometimes is that kids can hide themselves a bit, they can be much more independent because there's a lot of other things going on.

SAVILE: Looking back, one hundred per cent correct, nobody took any notice of me.

CLARE: But you seem to have had from very early on, as you describe it now, a sense of confidence in yourself.

SAVILE: Sure. Maybe I wasn't clever enough to be in trouble.

CLARE: How clever were you? Do you, have you any measure?

SAVILE: Academically? I went to a school where we didn't have exams, I went to a thing called an elementary school – you went in at four, came out at fourteen. There were no exams. You just moved up a class a year only because you grew out of the desk.

CLARE: But you know that cleverness also refers to an innate ability to think and achieve and so on. I saw somewhere, in fact it recurs in a lot of cuttings about you, an IQ figure which suggests that actually you do know that you're a damn clever man, because it's a high figure.

SAVILE: I've been in Mensa, a member of Mensa and I'm only a member of Mensa again because I was doing a programme with Mensa people, they liked the programme that I did with them and they said 'We want to make you an honorary member,' and I said 'I don't get honorary anything, I don't take honorary anything mate.'

CLARE: You mean I can't make you an honorary member of the Royal College of Psychiatrists, you're going to train the whole way through?

SAVILE: So therefore I said 'I'll go in for the exam, but clip my name off the top and if the assessors don't pass it I never took the exam in the first place,' that's the shrewd part of it, 'cos I wouldn't have the newspapers say he is thick, you understand. I don't care if I'm thick, it wasn't in my interests it be known. And so they did. So they photocopied my exam thing, clipped the top off and sent it to two assessors. One give me a hundred and fifty, one gave me a hundred and fifty-one, one hundred and forty-eight was the pass, so suddenly I was a member of Mensa.

CLARE: But you've said several times to me that maybe you aren't clever enough to have problems.

SAVILE: Could be, I don't know.

CLARE: What do you mean by that? Is that because you associate cleverness with having problems? Do you think that in fact clever people do tend to have problems?

SAVILE: I know a lot of professional people that would top themselves. I know a lot of people in your game that have topped themselves. Now then your game is what I call the brain game, and if they can organise other people's brains but they can't organise their own, and they top themselves up against a bannister or something like that, well it means of course there's something wrong. So therefore my simplicity said that maybe they were too clever. Maybe they could see things I can't see. I don't see problems, maybe they could see problems.

CLARE: Has anybody ever said that you're an unimaginative sort of chap?

SAVILE: No, but you can. It'll make no difference to me if you say I'm unimaginative, make no difference at all.

CLARE: Actually, in truth Jimmy, nothing I would say would make any difference to you?

SAVILE: Well, no 'cos you're a human being you see and it's your opinion. All I know is that after today I've got to go and do my thing in the world tomorrow. Question number one, am I doing my thing at the cost of somebody else? Answer, no. Am I doing my thing in getting plenty? Answer, yes. What am I doing with the plenty? Am I trying to put it about a little bit, including not so much what I've got as what time I've got? Answer, yes. Why do I put it about a little bit? I put it about a bit because obviously the good Lord has seen to it that I'm a bit lucky, right, for his own reasons, why, I don't know. Now if I'm a bit lucky I don't see any reason why I shouldn't spread it about a bit maybe, and make somebody else a bit lucky. Some poor sods who are down the road who for no fault of their own are finding it a bit hard. If I can give them a lift that's what, it's not yukky, you know it's not do-goodie, it's none of that crap game but it's nice simple stuff and I don't think there's anything wrong with it. It's a very simplistic way of going on. Maybe one of my problems for somebody like yourself is that I'm far too simple.

CLARE: Supposing I said to you, is there anything that you can imagine that would greatly disturb your life, that would break it up, that might make you a more churned up emotional person? For example, because you're very familiar with a place like Stoke Mandeville, how do you think you would cope, if God forbid, you tripped over something and broke your neck?

SAVILE: Don't know, don't know. I don't think I'd be a very good patient. I have seen what it costs to be a patient in terms of human fight. Now I don't know. I'd like to think that I had that fight, but I don't know, and that's why I come downstairs sideways because I'm very conscious of accidents now, so therefore I take inordinate care over many things. I haven't the faintest idea if I'd be very good or very bad. I'd cross that bridge when I came to it. I'd hope I'd be all right.

CLARE: But you have thought about it to the extent that you've modified your behaviour?

SAVILE: Oh yes, in exactly the same way as in the early discos, when people used to come in and they were a bit drugged up or a bit boozed up, I modified my behaviour then because I didn't want any part of that, even though I was the guv'nor. So I let them get on with it. I didn't say 'You are stupid.' If they asked me, if they said 'Do you think I'm stupid,' I'd say 'Yes you are.' But I wouldn't suddenly go out in some evangelical way and say 'I think that you are stupid for taking that.' It's not my game, you understand.

CLARE: That's fair enough. A related question – could you ever imagine yourself so depressed that you couldn't go on?

SAVILE: I'm sure that in the right circumstances, if the good Lord gives me fourteen hammer blows one after the other, all different ones, I'm sure that I would feel a lot different to what I feel now.

CLARE: What would hurt you most if you lost it, or if it was taken away from you?

SAVILE: Oh, freedom. I've got the freedom to do pretty well anything now including being bored, or being alone or being with people or getting things. I suppose if I didn't have that I would only see that as a temporary setback because somewhere my inventiveness is such that if I had everything taken away from me now it wouldn't be long before I got it back again. I've been skint once and I'm not skint now, but I ain't going to be skint no more.

CLARE: But freedom is important?

SAVILE: Well freedom, I'm trying to answer your question.

CLARE: You move quite a bit around. You're a mobile man. You don't put down roots.

SAVILE: No, not really, not really.

CLARE: You don't carry much baggage?

SAVILE: I've got a shoulder bag that has not been unpacked for nearly thirty years. It's a different bag when it wears out. But I mean I never unpack completely anything, anywhere, because I don't usually sleep in the same bed more than two nights running 'cos there's no point in it. I wander round like I sail the country.

CLARE: I'm wondering really what is it like to be someone who can say, as you did very commonsensically now, 'I'm really free, I could do almost anything.' Lots of poor sods, including me, struggling away we wonder, 'One day if I were free enough what would I do?' You are free enough.

SAVILE: Right. You're not in that world so therefore you don't know. You are constrained by certain things. I'm not in your world. I'm not constrained pretty well by anything. The tough thing in life is ultimate freedom, that's when the battle starts. Ultimate freedom is what it's all about, because you've got to be very strong to stand for ultimate freedom. Ask anybody who's ever won the pools and they'll say that their lives may have been better to a sense but they were far more complicated, right. Take any pop star who was nothing one day and suddenly was somebody with plenty of money the next day, it was marvellous for them, but it wasn't half complicated from what it used to be, right? Ultimate freedom is the big challenge. Now, I've got it, and I can tell you there's not many of us that have got ultimate freedom. With doing the things that I do, wearing the caps that I wear, I've got some considerable clout as well, all over, that is where the battle, the personal battle starts now. I would like to think that I've beaten that because I don't use my clout or coin or whatever for bad purposes. I prefer not to use them for any purposes but if anybody asks, then I can then produce an answer very often, so that's where the battle is. Now, ultimate freedom is what I should think, you tell me from a psychologist's point of view, ultimate freedom is what everybody would try to hope for eventually. And I've got news for you, it's like winning the pools. When you get it you've got to be very strong to handle it. I like to think if I actually said that I'm very strong, well only because I've managed to handle complete and ultimate utter freedom. It's marvellous but it's dangerous.

CLARE: Is it a battle for you? Are you conscious that there are things you have to resist that this freedom would enable you to do?

SAVILE: Yes, sure and do you know what helps me in the battle? My porter colleagues in my hospitals. I make oil and water mix. I still knock about with the people I was down the pit with. I still knock about with porters who are now retired that I've known, and if my ultimate freedom and money gave me any airs and graces they would soon have me down a peg or two. So they are very vital to me because we all of us don't really know how we are to other people before other people tell us. I've got a whole raft of people who've known me for all my life practically who would soon tell me if my feet ever started to leave the floor. So they're very useful to me, they're very vital to me.

CLARE: And that is one of the big dangers, that you'd develop airs and graces, that you'd become what you aren't?

SAVILE: Well, you would change, and I don't particularly want to change. So one of the battles, you're asking me about the battle of ultimate freedom, the battle of ultimate freedom is – is it going to change you for better, worse, or leave you alone? I like to think it's left me alone. But it would be easy to be corrupted by many things, when you've got ultimate freedom, especially when you've got clout. I could be corrupted. I'd like to think that up to press I've managed to stay like I was. I'm still acceptable to my low-income friends and they don't blame me for being lucky. They're cleverer than me, some of them, but they ain't as lucky as me, which is why they're skint and I'm loaded. And on the days that they get the hump that I'm loaded and they're not, then I'm as hard with them as they are with me. And I say 'Hey, don't you have a go at me for being lucky, if my number comes out of the bingo box, don't you shout at me pal. My number come out of the bingo box, yours hasn't, how do I know that my number isn't going to come out of the death box tomorrow or the accident box tomorrow, and how do you know your number's not coming out of the bingo box tomorrow. You could finish up well-loaded, I could finish up well-skint.' We don't know do we.

CLARE: Have you got to be always on your guard against being used?

SAVILE: No, that doesn't bother me in the slightest. Nobody uses me, I can see that coming a mile off. It just doesn't work that, doesn't bother me in the slightest, nobody uses me. They might think they might, I've got news for you pal, they've got to get up very early in the morning.

CLARE: Given this issue of ultimate freedom, there's nothing therefore that you want that you haven't got?

SAVILE: No I've got everything. Ask me, what I've got left in life.

CLARE: What have you got left in life?

SAVILE: To wake up tomorrow, 'cos if tomorrow is as good as today that'll do for me.

Tom Sharpe

Of all the interviews I have conducted *In the Psychiatrist's Chair* I have never laughed so much as I did during the one with Tom Sharpe. And yet in many ways it was one of the most distressing on account of the story he told of his extraordinary childhood, his malign, highly disturbed father, his experiences in South Africa and his long-standing psychological difficulties which despite all sorts of therapy have lasted all his life. The fact is that he has the most remarkable ability to take the ludicrousness, lunacy, the horror and the anguish of life and turn them into high comedy and farce. He is also equipped with the most mobile and humorous face – a slight droop of the lips or rumble of the voice and it is impossible to remain serious. This is yet another interview in which a father emerges as a powerful and in this case largely destructive influence. Tom Sharpe's account of him is compelling, insightful, humorous and ultimately forgiving. Yet it is a truly terrible story with a terrible legacy. To this day Tom Sharpe cannot go anywhere where there is a crowd and silence – church, cinema, theatre, underground train. If he does he experiences symptoms of panic and anxiety – physical sensations in his limbs, palpitations, dizziness, dry mouth, a dreadful feeling of panic bordering on terror and an almost irresistible urge to shout out obscenities. He has had all sorts of psychiatric treatment – psychoanalytic psychotherapy, behaviour therapy, anxiety-relieving drugs, relaxation therapy.

Sharpe feels an almost irresistible urge to vocalise obscenities but he has never actually done so. In general he avoids the potentially distressing situation – large, crowded, silent spaces. The duty of having to sit through his father's racist and fascist rantings in awesome church buildings as a small, frightened, angry boy seems to have created the culture medium for the seeding and growth of this particular neurosis. Doubtless the complex when it finally flowered was provoked by other factors but the result is a man deeply troubled by the issue of control. He does not feel in control of his feelings – the feeling of anger in particular. Rather he is driven by urges he does not recognise and cannot bend to his will. A recurrent dream – of being compelled to place the sun inside a billiard ball – echoes his predicament, his sense of being out of control.

The anxious and panicky individual who is afraid of his emotions is afraid of the things that arouse them. In compulsion neurosis, the influential psychoanalyst Otto Fenichel argued, thinking and talking gradually become substitutes for the emotions connected with reality. But they have to be handled with care for they are dangerous, almost magically so. A careless word might make effective the sadistic impulses that have been kept at bay with so much effort. In Tom Sharpe's case, it is not difficult to comprehend how the violent impulses arose, nor their likely target. Intense feelings are provoked by his father's behaviour. By a supreme effort, conscious and unconscious, such feelings are repressed. However, this repressed anxiety becomes displaced, giving way to an anxiety about words – that these will reveal the true aggressive feelings that have with such effort been controlled.

The sadistic aspect of obscene utterances is obvious enough. Tom Sharpe makes plain the nature of his aggressive feelings towards his father and indeed towards anything and everything that reminds him of patriarchal power, such as organised religion, traditional rituals, professional authority, political tyranny. The feared utterances, of course, are not merely aggressive but sexual as well. There is a sexual gain to be derived from uttering forbidden sexual words. Coprolalia, indulged or controlled, is often seen to be a matter of repressed libido. In a personal letter to me giving me permission to use the interview, Tom Sharpe hinted that the onset of his compulsion coincided with the start of an intense, forbidden sexual liaison.

What is of interest is the fact that Tom Sharpe has used the magic of words to express albeit in fictional and therefore sublimated terms much of the anger, aggression, ridicule and hatred which relate to his early relationship with his disturbed and disturbing father. In a succession of satirical novels, he savages the cruelty and lunacy of a racist, fascist, fundamentalist apartheid system, a system of which his father might well have approved and the petty obsessions and compulsions of academic life which have been grandly and pathologically elaborated into revered Oxbridge traditions.

Tom Sharpe has not found psychiatric treatment of much use although he has tried various forms. Obsessional impulses are often difficult to treat particularly if they occur in the setting of severe anxiety, are continually reinforced by stressful experiences and afflict a particularly obsessional personality. I don't know because I did not ask how obsessional in other ways Sharpe is – whether he is particularly pedantic, meticulous, perfectionist, punctual, whether he finds making a decision an agony, whether he is rigid and inflexible in his views, whether high moral standards are exaggerated to become painful guilty preoccupations with wrong-doing. People with obsessional personalities commonly lack a sense of humour. In Tom Sharpe's case it is his most obvious and attractive feature.

Perhaps too many doctors and therapists remind him of his father, spouting their nonsense with the same degree of self-importance and lack of insight. In his letters to me, he does not conceal his humorous contempt for most of my professional colleagues. He remains afflicted, yet a writer of some of the funniest contemporary prose in the English language. Whether these two facets of the man are crucially connected I do not know. Nor does he. It is, however, some consolation to him to know that had he had a different father, perhaps a man of sanity, wisdom and compassion, he Thomas Ridley Sharpe, might have grown up to become something predictable, secure and orthodox – a vicar perhaps or even a psychiatrist. As it is he has been able to transform his angry, aggressive, wounded feelings into biting, satirical prose and many hundreds of thousands of readers are the beneficiaries.

CLARE: Thomas Ridley Sharpe was born in 1928, his mother was South African, his father a unitarian clergyman from

Northumberland. Tom Sharpe was educated at Lancing College and then at Cambridge University, did his National Service with the Royal Marines and in the 1950s he worked in South Africa as a social worker, a teacher and a photographer. In 1961, when he sued a right-wing newspaper for libel he was deported from South Africa. After his return to England he spent ten years as a lecturer in history and became a full-time novelist in 1971. Since then he has published a number of best-selling novels, two of them, *Porterhouse Blues* and *Blot On The Landscape*, have been adapted for television, while a film based on his comic anti-hero Henry Wilt was recently released. Thomas Sharpe, do you spend much time thinking about yourself and what has made you what you are?

SHARPE: Yes, I think I probably do, well, I'm certainly puzzled.

CLARE: By what in particular?

SHARPE: Well, I mean my attitudes are, they're not, when I say normal, they're not the usual ones, I don't think, and certainly I don't understand the world, I don't make any pretence of doing so. If you're an almost unconscious comic novelist or writer you have to be a bit puzzled as to why, what influences brought this about. I suppose in the worst possible way you'd say you were self-absorbed, or I would say that I was self-absorbed, I don't know.

CLARE: When you look at your life, do you identify a really powerful influence for good or ill?

SHARPE: Well actually for good and ill, which it was really, it was clearly my father. He was a relatively old man when I was born. He was fifty-six when I was born, so that now I'm sixty-three I'd have a seven-year-old child hanging around. All my brothers, brothers and sisters, were much older, and here was a man on the verge of retirement really, living in Croydon. He himself had been mind-blown by the events that had taken place in his life. I mean he was a Victorian, he was born in 1872 and there's no question whatsoever that he was the most powerful influence in my life and in some respects it was accidentally good. The spin-off was good, but I think in fact that the actual influence was a terrible one (terrible?) oh yes a terrible one. But you see I don't believe in blaming one's parents for the simple reason that they themselves were the product of environments which, well, even a son of my age can't understand. He was one of a very large family. My grandfather was a quarryman at the time and they gave, I don't think this was probably uncommon, they gave my father away to a maiden aunt who had a little bit of money. My father, he had to work during the summer, I know he's always reckoned that he was small because he worked in a glass-blowing factory when he was fourteen, and he was a beer runner for some iron foundry and he worked down mines. He did all these things. He was such a Victorian, and then his first wife died and I think my father nearly had a nervous breakdown. At one stage he was sent by his congregation, he was then in Manchester, to recover from this, one of his breakdowns, they all got together and they raised the money for the Reverend Sharpe and they sent him off to South America on this ship. Well, four days out of Liverpool, it was a coal ship, it caught fire and my father recounted, rather joyfully, how he used to walk the deck when it was red hot, and this was supposed to be a cure for his nerves! He was a very nervous man. Anyway he never got the respect in this country because he didn't have a degree or anything of that sort, so he always had a chip on his shoulder. He felt that he could have done better, you know, and he went to Germany in 1928, the year I was born, and from that moment onwards he became a national socialist. Fundamentally he was a pacifist, he didn't want another war. And yet he was taken in and at the same time there was his anti-semitism, there can be no doubt about that.

CLARE: You can remember it?

SHARPE: Oh yes, only too well. He regarded Mosley as left-wing! He belonged to the Imperial Fascist League and the Nordic League which was violently anti-semitic and foul, I mean really vile. He belonged to the right club and he had a friend called Joyce and he used to say to my mother, 'I think I'll go out and see Joyce tonight,' you know, and I was about ten and I thought this was a bit odd, mother doesn't seem to mind him going out with this girl. And of course it was William Joyce who was later Lord Haw-Haw and who was hanged after the war for broadcasting. And I remember seeing Joyce in the house once. It was the only time he ever came, because my mother kicked up such a fuss about that one. So father was a very strong influence. He was a frightening man actually too because of his irritations and that's something I've inherited from him too.

CLARE: Frightening in the explosive sense?

SHARPE: Oh yes, in the explosive sense and the beatings one got.

CLARE: He was violent? Or could be?

SHARPE: Oh he was, and in those days it was common, I mean, you know, working-class fathers and so on, you know, all right he might be a minister, yes . . .

CLARE: And effectively of course you were the youngest in this family, the other children by this stage would have to some extent grown away?

SHARPE: Oh yes, and I think in a sense they probably had it worse, I know my real brother did, he had it far worse than I did, because I think my father had mellowed by the time I came along. But what he did, you see, he used to walk me to school and talk about Plato. My head was filled with astonishing sort of stuff at a very early age and I mean I read the, I mean that awful forgery called, you know *The Protocols of Zion* and the filthy things like *The Father of Lies*, full of horrors, full of executions. I think frankly poor old father, he didn't have a clue how to bring children up. That's the simple way of putting it. He didn't. He hadn't got a clue.

CLARE: Did it give you nightmares? Do you remember being troubled by it?

SHARPE: Oh yes, I can remember a nightmare that I had. I had a frightful nightmare actually. It gives me the willies to think about it now. I was faced with a problem. I had a task of putting the sun inside a pingpong ball. The mind is such a very peculiar organ that it can come up with that one because

I hadn't thought of it. You've got space. You've got 93 million miles to cross of empty space with not a breath of air. You have the fact that when you get near the sun you're going to be roasted. And worst of all, you've got the size of the sun which is gigantic, and you've got the pingpong ball which is very small. The pingpong ball's made of celluloid which explodes into flame. I mean what a conundrum! What a frightful thing to have to do and in a dream world you do have to do things. It's not as though you've got a choice and say, 'well hang on a moment, let's be reasonable about this.' So that was a nightmare which I've never been able to explain.

CLARE: Did you feel that your father had expectations of you?

SHARPE: Oh yes he did.

CLARE: What did he want you to do?

SHARPE: At one stage we were walking down Selsdon Road in Croydon and he was talking about the need for dictators! He wanted me to be a genius, that's another thing he definitely did. He wanted in fact, oh the expectations were gigantic and they were silly.

CLARE: And in the midst of all this what was your mother like? What was happening to her, a much younger woman?

SHARPE: She had a good sense of humour, but it was a dry one and my mother on her death bed – you might want to take this out, but I'll tell you all the same. First of all it was an Irish nurse, a matron who rang me up and said your mother's dying, so I go over there and mother's dying. She's eighty-seven. She's got a kidney failure, she's in no pain or anything, she's no glasses, no teeth, you know *sans* anything and along comes this woman and she said, 'Come on me darlin',' she said to my mother. And my mother doesn't even open her eyes but she said, 'I'm not your darling,' she said, 'I'm Mrs Sharpe.' Now I respect that. But that's tough, she's not going to take any nonsense, she never did. I don't think she was a very nice woman. I don't know. I mean she was nice enough to me but I think she was also herself. I think she had a hard life and she stuck by my father when she shouldn't have. Father was interesting. The point was that life was lively and he, he was a wonderful speaker, and he had an enormous amount of charm, you see, outside the home.

CLARE: Did he resent you? This after-thought?

SHARPE: Oh, I have letters which indicate that, yes, he did. I've got actually some letters, the only letters I've got 'cos mother burnt everything of his, including his sermons.

CLARE: And how did your mother cope with this man?

SHARPE: I don't know what bitterness there was underneath, there was a lot of bitterness after he died.

CLARE: Did she protect you?

SHARPE: Mmmn, tried to.

CLARE: She knew what was going on?

SHARPE: Oh well, there wasn't abuse in the sense of hole-in-corner stuff.

CLARE: You say you have much of that in you.

SHARPE: I have a foul temper yes.

CLARE: Still?

SHARPE: Mmn.

CLARE: When we were talking about your father you, you thought he'd had good and bad influences on you.

SHARPE: Well yes, I mean he was wrong, I mean he died in 1944 in March. He could go on in his dream world, this platonic universe of his, you see, the republic where you had an elite you know and this was his philosophical justification for Nazism, all this racial twaddle and he'd go on believing it, in fact, and he did believe right till the end, right through the war.

CLARE: He saw the war as a great mistake presumably?

SHARPE: Oh, an absolute, terrible mistake, you know, we should have been backing the Germans against the Russians. The evil lay in Bolshevism.

CLARE: Would he have said any of this stuff in his sermons?

SHARPE: He did!

CLARE: In his unitarian church?

SHARPE: Yes, I sat behind a man and watched his neck getting redder and redder and redder in Ealing, oh yes, he, he, oh yes, he said it!

CLARE: Did anybody ever protest about it?

SHARPE: My God, there were rows, yes. I remember very well sitting behind this bloke and his neck (laugh) you know he went absolutely puce. By God he was angry, but you know he didn't leap to his feet and say, 'You're talking twaddle,' which he should have done.

CLARE: What did your father die of?

SHARPE: He died of pneumonia. He went for a walk on a Saturday and he got caught in the rain without a jacket and he was seventy-two and he came home and he got the 'flu and they hadn't got antibiotics and he died on the Monday.

CLARE: Can you remember your feelings?

SHARPE: Oh yes, I can remember them. I certainly wasn't sorry. There may be a shock situation, a moment when in fact you feel rather good before anything else hits you! I didn't attend the funeral. My mother didn't want that. She had him buried in an unmarked grave.

CLARE: What was his relationship with your mother like? I mean how much of this was sort of sexual frustration that he lived his life outside the home.

SHARPE: I don't know how well they got on, in fact, 'cos when my grandfather came over in 1922 from South Africa he said to my mother 'I'm going to take you home,' and she refused, so I think there must have been something very wrong at that stage.

CLARE: She told you this?

SHARPE: Oh, well yes it was known, definitely. The whole family knew that. The South Africans knew it. They were shocked and she always regretted in fact that she hadn't done that.

CLARE: You said at the very beginning that you sometimes think your attitudes to things are not normal, that was the word you used.

SHARPE: Well, I think if you've got a bizarre sense of humour you are looking at things in a peculiar way and, there-fore, that's what I meant by not normal. I mean I sort of flipped, I mean I didn't have a nervous breakdown, at least it wasn't a breakdown, a full-blown one, but I developed symptoms, when I was seventeen, coming up for eighteen.

CLARE: What happened?

SHARPE: Well, it happened in church. I don't know why on earth I was taken to church early on to sit through father's sermons which went on for forty-five minutes sometimes, you can imagine, frightful things. Anyway one day I'm in Lancing chapel which is a very, enormous chapel. I don't know if you know it, it's 172 feet high, it's a school chapel, you know, it's like a bloody cathedral and there's this rather nice chap who was nattering away, he was giving a sermon, and I suddenly had this awful experience which I still get. I mean I can't go to church, I can't go to anything where there's silence, where there's a crowd and where there's silence. I cannot do that. It just you know came up my legs, that's the way it comes – Zzoooppp, and the urge to scream, you know scream obscenities, you know, absolute, anything, things that you didn't even know, but you'd just read about (laugh) they were self-abasing I can tell you. (Laugh) I mean you know, if you're ever in an Underground train and it stops and you see a bloke in the corner shivering that's me, 'cos nobody ever talks in those Undergrounds. You know when the damn thing stops and there's Sharpe wondering if he's going to blurt out some obscenity. Even now at sixty-three, and there are lots of people in the world who are like this you know, poor devils, that's possibly one of the reasons I came on this programme, but it's, you know, La Tourette Syndrome. I wondered if I didn't have, something like that. It was psychologically induced.

CLARE: You never had a tic?

SHARPE: No, I never had a tic, but I had this, this terrible urge, you see.

CLARE: Did you ever do it, did you ever vocalise it?

SHARPE: No, no, I never did. Somebody once said to me, what have you been on? I've been on every damn drug there is under the sun. As for suing drug companies for their wretched pills, I believe in them. In certain circumstances they are a great help and I hope to God I'm never taken off them.

CLARE: These are tranquillisers we're talking about.

SHARPE: Yes, they're tranquillisers and they're anti-anxiety ones. It was panic attack you see came on, whoop.

CLARE: With your hearting beating fast?

SHARPE: Oh everything (and feeling dizzy) yes, the whole lot . . . (mouth going dry) . . . terrible. It comes up your leg, a sort of wave you see, I don't know why.

CLARE: Coupled with a terrible apprehension?

SHARPE: Well, that you're going to do it, yes of course. But I mean if you've got father up there and he happens to be God, which I assume that must be what it's about, I don't know, nobody does, I mean you're not the only shrink I've met believe me (laugh) . . .

CLARE: Have you met many?

SHARPE: Oh yes, dozens of them. I had to when I was at Cambridge, I couldn't go to lectures you see, because there again there was bloody God sitting down there, he was bleating on. He was usually lying anyway.

CLARE: But you never actually vocalised it . . . It was just this terror that you might in those certain circumstances?

SHARPE: And it's still there, it's silly to say it's not.

CLARE: Are there situations you now avoid? (yes absolutely) You wouldn't go to church. Any other things you wouldn't go to, would you go to the theatre?

SHARPE: No, very seldom, I mean we don't want to go into every phobic thing. There are a whole damn lot of them, I mean what the hell do you do, you've got to laugh, you know . . .

CLARE: Did you ever go to a psychiatrist for long-term therapy?

SHARPE: Oh yes, I mean I had more Jungian therapy than . . . I didn't have any money, I used to motorcycle all the way down to Durban and had, I had Jung, Jung, Jung!

CLARE: And did it help?

SHARPE: Well, you see the glory of your profession as a matter of fact . . . Well you're not a psychoanalyst so I mean you can actually see what the effects are, but I mean a psychoanalyst is in a wonderful position of being able to say, 'Well, if you hadn't had it you know you would be much worse.' I even went down to your, I think it was your place was it, the Maudsley. I don't want to give you all my phobias because it gets borings for the listeners and so on. I mean it makes me sound as an absolute bag of nonsense, which I am (laugh). It isn't self-pity. You've got to live with this damn thing. You know far worse things happen in the world, so you just can avoid most of these things. Anyway, I lay there and they said 'Now this is definitely going to work; now all you've got to do is imagine yourself in a situation.' I could imagine myself in the situation no end!

CLARE: And then they relaxed you? They tried to relax you, did they?

SHARPE: I couldn't get into a state of anxiety imagining it, there was no way.

CLARE: It had to be the real thing?

SHARPE: It had to be the real thing, yes, so there wasn't any use my doing that. I couldn't then sort of learn to breathe and relax down from that situation.

CLARE: How crippling was it? You got through Cambridge.

SHARPE: Oh yes, it is, it is pretty crippling.

CLARE: Yes, even now?

SHARPE: Oh yes, it is indeed, oh yes, very. It is crippling and there's no question about that at all. I mean there are certain things I simply cannot do.

CLARE: When did you realise that you had this interesting way of looking at the world? At university?

SHARPE: No, no, no. Really when I began to write that infernal book, I mean the first book, *Riotous Assembly* which is about South Africa and it suddenly took off into this sort of bizarre world which actually was hysterically funny but it was a horrible world.

CLARE: How did you come to start the writing?

SHARPE: Well, I was writing in South Africa all the time, writing plays and so on. I got married again in 1969 and my wife went back to the States 'cos she was only over here on holiday and I sat down to write a story and, a serious one, and suddenly it took off into this wild farce.

CLARE: Had you ever written farce before?

SHARPE: Never, never, no. The farce sprang from the logic of the situation and the logic of the situation is that apartheid is mad and once you start talking about people who are black as though they were not people, well, it is hysterical because in fact something's gone mad. The other thing I was sick to death, too, of middle-class people in South Africa writing middle-class novels about the moral torments of white people or black people. This wasn't where it's at as the modern expression is, where it's at is a sort of, another awful expression, interface between a whole lot of ignorant white cops and ordinary black people trying to go about their business, and getting themselves raped, you know not getting themselves raped, but *being* raped and shot and drowned. I mean the torture that went on in South Africa in police stations regularly, I mean a regular thing. I've got a cutting from the *Guardian* within the last ten years in which a magistrate said, 'Well how did you get a confession out of this bloke? You say he signed a confession.' The policeman said, 'Well the usual method.' And the magistrate said, 'Well, what is the usual method?' He said 'Well, we stuck his head in a bucket of water until he nearly drowned.' That's a policeman in a magistrates court in Capetown! So this was a standard. What sort of world are we living in where this is normal, where a policeman can say this is a normal method?

CLARE: And *Porterhouse Blues*, where did that come out of?

SHARPE: I only got to Cambridge really because of the 1944 Education Act. Well, first of all I was educated during the war when you didn't get much of an education, and particularly when you were planning to be, you know an SS man!

CLARE: Were you?

SHARPE: Yes, I was. I was planning to be. I was looking forward to this heroic role. I didn't know what it entailed, mind you, but (laugh) I just thought the uniform great. Anyway one went up to university with vast expectations and a great deal of nervousness, because you know, as I've said, I didn't come from the right class. I was the first person who'd ever been to university in my family, and I wasn't intellectually equipped in any case to meet all these dreadful old dons. You know, it was a very bizarre experience, I found it was anyway.

CLARE: It seemed a crazy world too?

SHARPE: Well it did, and especially if you've got this terrible urge to get up in the middle of every lecture you're supposed to go to and yell. So you can't go to lectures you know, what the hell do you do? You go and see a psychiatrist in Grantchester and you take your exams on sodium amytal, I mean sodium amytal is not the great stimulant that people should be having when they do a tripos! You've got double vision for one thing and the sort of doses that I was taking to get into that damn room with 800 other students.

CLARE: Was when you saw the psychiatrist in Cambridge one of the first times that you started to go over this childhood experience? When would somebody from my profession have started to take an interest in you and your father for example? Was it then?

SHARPE: Well yes, well probably, I went to see a man called Davis, I think he was a professor, was it Davis? Anyway I remember what he did. He was wonderful, splendid fellow actually. I'd attended one of his lectures on how you created neuroses in rats or cats it was actually, cats, phenobaritone in large enough doses gives cats neuroses, bad ones I gather. Another way of doing it is just when they're about to eat some grub and they're getting very hungry is to give an air blast down the back of the neck. So I sat through this lecture. I did sit through that one at the back by the door, anyway. I thought this man was obviously the cure, he was going to get all the answers for me, and I remember this wretched fellow (laugh) looking at me and he said, 'What sort of a degree do you want to get?' I said, 'Well I'd like to get a first.' He said, 'Really?' He said, 'Well, I think you ought to know straightaway that you're not capable, intellectually capable, of getting a first.' It was blunt and it was to the point, but if he'd said, 'Get the hell out of university,' it would have been fine. I mean it wouldn't have been fine, but what he actually said was no help for one's morale. If he'd said, 'Look you might get a decent 2/2 or you know an upper,' you know or, 'Frankly my dear fellow go and play a bit of golf, and just get the degree you can get,' if only he'd said that. But no, no, he had to do this other one, and I remember the Dean of Pembroke, this is somewhat later, when a fellow committed suicide and I remember him saying, 'Well of course he was hopeless, hopeless, hopeless fellow, he should have been sent down last year as a matter of fact, dreadful really, should have been sent down.' Well, as a degree of sympathy for the bloke who'd gone and gassed himself . . . I put this into the Dean of Porterhouse, you know where he says, 'We haven't had a decent suicide lately.' I remember there was a terrible scandal in Trinity. It wasn't that a fellow killed himself, quite a reasonable thing to do apparently, no the fact was he drank sherry out of a tumbler! He might have been using one of these plastic cups and this was regarded as so infra dig, this was, he went down in history. This was a fellow in Trinity, who practically had to take to his room! And if only he'd used a glass it would have been all right (laugh). You see where hysteria comes in. You want to help. You write to his parents, say, 'Very sorry about little Johnny. It's a great sorrow to us all, but his table manners weren't of the best — (laugh). I had a friend who used to run for the Drag Hunt, you know, used to send a bag of sawdust down to the zoo and a panther would piss on it obediently and they'd sent it back and they'd tie it round this fellow's waist and he'd run you see and then after a while these other fellows on horse-back, you see, who could afford horses, they'd come belting after him. But one day he didn't get far enough, so the ruddy hounds were on top of him and you know this fellow raised his crop at him. It was a Winchetser bloke who raised his crop! Well, this was the atmosphere. This is the Cambridge that I knew in a sense. I wasn't any good at sport as you can imagine 'cos I couldn't run or do anything like that, and I wasn't bright enough to be an arty-crafty, I was a sort of in-betweener really. 'Sharpe yes, it's a great pity that he ever came.' (laugh).

CLARE: And then you had this affliction.

SHARPE: And then, yes, then I had an affliction.

CLARE: Your colleagues around that time, what would they have made of you? Do you enjoy making people laugh?

SHARPE: Yes I do, and I enjoy laughing, I enjoy conversation, I think that's the one thing that I really do. I can say that I enjoy most of all listening to people. I mean it's a two-way thing.

CLARE: We were talking earlier about your smoking. Did you always smoke?

SHARPE: No, I learnt that in the Marines, you were supposed to get fit in the Marines and they used to give you twenty fags for eightpence halfpenny, very good fags they were too, at the end of every hour. We used to, we spent six months doing square bashing. This was after the war. We would go on a pre-war marine training which was six months' drill, six months' drill and at the end of every hour they'd say five minutes' break for smoking. Well, there wasn't an awful lot else to do, 'cos you're going to bash up and down that wretched parade ground again, so you smoked and my father was a smoker, tremendous smoker. So this was a thing I enjoyed enormously.

CLARE: When did you give it up?

SHARPE: On September 15th 1987.

CLARE: You remember the date?

SHARPE: Oh, only too well, yes.

CLARE: Why, what happened?

SHARPE: Well, I had angina. I was in Spain and I had this strange pain in the middle of my chest in a television programme. Well, I knew it was a bit odd because it was spreading out. Well, I'm not a fool and I'm a sufficient hypochondriac if you want to know, to know that this is what heart attacks begin with, they've only got to go down the left arm and you're really . . . So they're taping all this stuff and I have a very lovely Spanish lady sitting opposite me who didn't speak a word of English and she had a female interpreter and I had a bearded man with a big paunch shouting through a piece in my ear, and you know there she was saying 'There's a lot of sex in your book,' and he was saying in my ear, this fat man with a beard saying, 'There's an awful lot of violence in your book,' and the pain began to get worse and worse and worse but I wasn't sweating you see and I could breathe, so I wasn't too worried. But at the end of it all it was really very painful indeed so I said, when they'd finished, they'd better call the doctor. By this time I was obviously ill. And so while we were waiting for the doctor they said, 'Well, why didn't you say it before?' I thought, well actually it was partly true you see. Well, it was all being taped I said, and I had the consolation of knowing, were I to pop off just now my daughters when they got married would be able to say to their husbands when they got very angry with them, let's put the video in and watch daddy dying again shall we? Well the Spanish were appalled at this (laugh). Anyway then the doctor came. The pain was really rather nasty, I was trying to take my mind off it. Anyway, that's all that was. Anyway they diagnosed angina and said no more snuff.

CLARE: You used to take snuff?

SHARPE: Yes, about a pound a month. Mind you I did smoke pipes at the same time and inhale, I mean I did everything wrong.

CLARE: Did you take the snuff off the back of your hand?

SHARPE: No no between my thumb and forefinger.

CLARE: Yes, what did it do for you?

SHARPE: Well, it had a chemical affect on the brain. It does. There's no question about this, and I've spoken to a number of people who've given up smoking and they all of them say that they don't have the mental stimulation. It's the nicotine. If you could have nicotine in a harmless form I'd go back to it, but you can't. And my doctor said, 'I've never met a fellow like you before,' he said, 'You know you've stopped smoking just like a shot, no complaints,' he said. I said 'You've never met a coward before have you?' He said, 'Willpower.' I said 'No willpower.' If the choice is smoking or dying you don't smoke, simple isn't it?

CLARE: Given that you saw a lot of psychiatrists about it, just going back for the last time to that extraordinary sense of tension and the feeling that you're going to explode and vocalise and so on, you were given various explanations and you met various psychiatrists, Jungians and behaviourists and classic pharmacologists who gave you drugs and so on, what's your understanding of it? What do you see, what makes most sense to you? What is the explanation that here you are, periodically in those kind of settings, charged up? . . .

SHARPE: Oh quite obviously, I think there is a powerful instinctive urge to be yourself, whatever that self is. There is, nevertheless, there's an element in the individual which says, 'I'm me and I'm jolly well going to do what I want, and I want to say things.' And I think that living in a Victorian home, because my father who was twenty-eight after all in 1900 and so was a Victorian, and I was born in 1928, another twenty-eight years so my father was fifty-six you know, a man who'd lived for twenty-eight years of his life in a very, very restricted religious atmosphere, a Methodist you know, and who really believed in paternalism, and where children, you know, made no noises. I remember playing so clearly you know 'cos we didn't kneel, we didn't have kneelers in the unitarian church, but everybody bent down and I used to play with the hymn books in the pews while he blathered on up there. Well, frankly I think it's a very natural thing for me to say, 'Oh for God's sake shut up!' and just yell obscenities or yell, I mean that seems to me what, you know, a child should have done. I think it was extremely stupid of my parents to have put me in that situation. You see that's the point, I think that's where this sort of came from and it was a rebuttal. It was an explosion against him and against if you like what he represented, standing in that pulpit and talking rubbish.